DARK BLUE

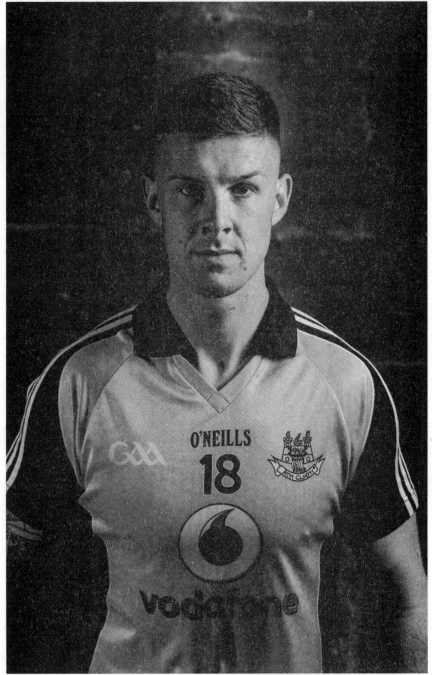

Born in 1994, Shane Carthy lives in the seaside town of Portmarnock in north Dublin. He has played Gaelic football at the very highest level, representing Dublin at Minor, U21 and Senior levels, and collecting five All Ireland medals to date. When he's not playing football, Shane spends most of his time with family and friends and travels the length and breadth of the country sharing his experiences with mental health.

DARK BLUE

THE DESPAIR BEHIND THE GLORY — MY JOURNEY BACK FROM THE EDGE

SHANE CARTHY

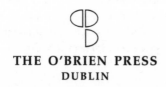

THE O'BRIEN PRESS
DUBLIN

First published 2021 by The O'Brien Press Ltd,
12 Terenure Road East, Rathgar, Dublin 6, D06 HD27, Ireland.
Tel: +353 1 4923333; Fax: +353 1 4922777
E-mail: books@obrien.ie. Website: www.obrien.ie
The O'Brien Press is a member of Publishing Ireland.

ISBN: 978-1-78849-150-1

Text © Shane Carthy 2021
Editing, typesetting, layout, design © The O'Brien Press Ltd

Front cover and inside photograph by Andres Poveda.
Cover and inside design by Emma Byrne.

8 7 6 5 4 3 2 1
25 24 23 22 21

Printed and bound by ScandBook AB, Lithuania.
The paper in this book is produced using pulp from managed forests.

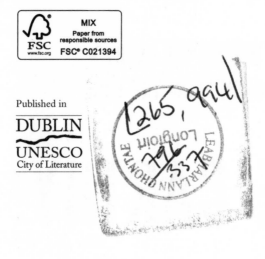

Published in

DUBLIN

UNESCO
City of Literature

Dedication

To all of those who are suffering in silence, in the hope that these words might help the light to shine in.

CONTENTS

CHAPTER I

MY YOUNGER YEARS

I grew up in Portmarnock, a beautiful seaside town in north County Dublin. Apart from its beach, Portmarnock is probably best known for its world-class golf course. Portmarnock Golf Club has hosted many tournaments, including the 1960 Canada Cup, the 1991 Walker Cup and the Irish Open on many occasions.

My parents, Angela and Gerry, cast me, along with my three sisters Stephanie, Mairead and Michelle, into every sport possible. We were known as the 'sporting mad' family. I guess that all stemmed from my dad, who was hugely involved in sport. From a very young age, he was in love with Gaelic, soccer and hurling. In fact, he even missed his own brother's wedding so that he could play a soccer match for his boyhood club, Glasnevin FC.

My mam was always very much into staying active too, playing badminton in the local Portmarnock Sport & Leisure club. My mam is a typical mother – family-orientated and kind-hearted, exuding warmth and caring. My dad has a slightly rougher exterior; he is hard-working, driven and disciplined by nature, and this rubbed off on my sisters and myself from early on. Whenever we started into something, he would say, 'Anything you do, do it to the best of your ability.'

My parents tell me I had so much energy as a kid that they were running out of sports to get me involved in. While I loved any sport I took up, two in particular gave me huge joy and satisfaction – Gaelic and soccer. Naomh Mearnóg GAA club and Portmarnock FC were the local sports clubs that nurtured the raw talent I had, starting at a very young age.

The GAA mini leagues were where my potential in Gaelic football was first spotted. This involved over 150 kids from the ages of four to seven, being coached in the fundamentals of Gaelic football. Even at the tender age of seven, Gerry Davey, who was my first underage manager, remarked to my parents that he saw 'something special' in me. My love for the game grew from there.

I attended my local primary school, St Marnock's, and my sporting ambition became apparent on Sports Day every year. From third to sixth class, in particular, there was a bit more riding on it – the prize was to be crowned sports boy/girl of the year. In third class, I had a burning desire to become sports boy of the year. So much so, that in the lead-up to Sports Day, I would visualise myself running across the line in first place in each race I entered.

On the day, my mam brought along a packet of Jaffa Cakes, Winegums and a bottle of Lucozade, to make sure my energy levels were brimming come the start of every race. Mam would later do this for school matches too – I recall her often bringing up a large bowl of pasta for me to eat on the way to a match.

With my dad's words of wisdom, 'Anything you do, do it to the best of your ability,' ringing in my ears, I was doing whatever it took to win. And it paid off – I was declared junior sports boy of the year, defeating my class-mates and the year above me too. The following year, I repeated this feat, and in fifth class, I was crowned senior sports boy of the year. One final push in my final year of primary school would win me the four-in-a-row, something that had never been done before.

As I went into my final Sports Day, there was a certain air of inevitably about things. As the first race was about to begin, my mam recalls hearing another classmate's mother saying, 'Mark said to me this morning, what's the point in racing? Shane Carthy is going to win anyway.'

This comment illustrates how my classmates saw me at the time – I seemed like an untouchable figure, who had everything going for him. This image was further enhanced when I went ahead and won again – school sports boy of the year, an unprecedented fourth year in a row.

I think I should point out at this stage that although I was achieving all of this success, I was never one to gloat about it. I was, and would like to think I still am, a very humble person. Although I like to keep myself to myself and stay away from the limelight, this was quickly becoming more difficult. My talent was being recognised by more and more people, par-ticularly in the Gaelic football world.

My dream from a very young age was to represent Dublin in Gaelic football, and at Easter of sixth class, I was given that opportunity. I was one of hundreds of footballers, from almost every club in Dublin, invited along to a trial in Raheny GAA club. We played a number of matches, and coaches chose who would go forward to the next trial. I was chosen for the second trial, among others in the group. Following this, coaches deliberated again on who they wanted.

Exactly a week following the second trial, I heard news back – I was one of the lucky few who had been chosen to represent Dublin in the upcoming Easter tournament. I was the only person picked from my school or my area, so this was a pretty big deal. I was selected as captain for the tournament and, as if things couldn't get any better, we won. This is where I began my Dublin career – in a small capacity, yes, but it was a start nonetheless.

I vividly remember sitting in the back left corner of Mr Greene's classroom on the Monday morning, as my friends asked what I had got up to at the weekend. I didn't want to gloat, but in fairness I was proud of what I had done, so I told them – I had captained the Dublin team in the Easter Gaelic tournament, and we won. The pedestal my peers regarded me as being on grew larger still.

CHAPTER 2

SECONDARY SCHOOL

In September 2007, I began attending my local secondary school, Portmarnock Community School. The transition from primary to secondary school can be an intimidating prospect for some, but for me it was seamless. I was lucky to know a few friends from primary school to start off with, and it didn't take me long to find more.

I got involved in almost every sport the school had to offer – Gaelic, soccer, hurling, athletics, you name it! This allowed me to quickly make new friends. I wasn't the most self-assured of people, but sport seemed to bring out a certain confidence in me. To be honest, approaching someone in class or on the corridors intimidated me, but during or after a bout of exercise I wouldn't have had a moment's hesitation, so this was where my friendships began. I soon found that people weren't shy in approaching me, perhaps wanting to be in with the guy who was 'good at anything he tried his hand at'.

One sport that I tried my hand at in first year was golf. My interest in the sport started when I found myself out in my back field one day with my friend Conor, who'd brought along a golf club and ball. He handed over the club and I swung at the ball. After a few aimless swipes into thin air, the club head made contact and the ball went soaring off into the distance. At that moment, my passion for the game of golf was born.

My parents weren't convinced that I'd stick at it, saying 'it's too slow a game for you'. I started off small, joining the local pitch and putt club. By January of first year, I had my own set of golf clubs and was a member of Malahide Golf Club.

This by no means meant that my love for other sports fell by the wayside, especially Gaelic football and soccer. In fact, in the same month that I joined Malahide Golf Club, I joined Malahide FC too. This team played in the Dublin District Schoolboys' League, regarded by many as the best league in the country. Many young boys dream of becoming a professional footballer, and I was no different. I just happened to be juggling a lot of dreams, including also playing with the Dublin senior footballers.

As if my stock couldn't grow any more in my first year at secondary school, I ended it off by picking up player of the year in the first year Gaelic football team at the school sports awards. First year was another building block in the ever-growing pedestal that people saw me as standing on.

As I headed into second year, I decided to narrow my sporting focus somewhat. I would concentrate on Gaelic and soccer, though I also kept up a bit of golf and pitch and putt. I continued to excel on the sporting field, captaining my club and school Gaelic teams that year. Captains are notorious for being extremely vocal, but I didn't quite fit this mould. There were no rousing speeches from me before games, and even out on the field you'd hardly hear a peep out of me. Neither my school nor club manager demanded this from me – they simply wanted 'my feet to do the talking'.

My club manager at the time, James Gahan, took me aside early on in the season. He always had a knack for saying the right things when they were needed, especially with me. I didn't mind captaining the team, but a part of me thought I was taking the opportunity away from someone else who could play the role better. James could sense this, and he told me, 'I don't think you realise the respect the lads have for you. All I want you to do this season is play football, and the rest will follow.' I guess this was an example of how my teammates and friends saw me – as a person to look up to and aspire to be like. I didn't want any of that, but because of a natural talent for sport, this was where I was.

The summer of second year arrived. While most people my age were down at the beach socialising, gathered around in a field or attending house parties, I wasn't doing any of those things. I was either at the Gaelic, golf or pitch and putt club, honing the skills I was learning. The work I was doing was paying off too. I once again represented Dublin at various events throughout the summer. My focus was very much on Gaelic and soccer, with golf being something I enjoyed on the side.

It simply wasn't in my nature to be happy with just being okay at something I was doing. I realised that I might not reach the top level in everything I did, but it wouldn't be through lack of trying. So, with school finished up for the summer, I spent hours on end up on the range in Malahide Golf Club, determined to continue improving my game. By the summer's end, the work I'd put in had paid dividends, as I was awarded Juvenile Golfer of the Year. You can imagine how my stock rose once again. As I sat back down on my seat having received the award, my friend Philip remarked, 'Is there anything you can't do?'

I entered my Junior Certificate year. The only things on my mind though were sport-related. I continued to play Gaelic, soccer, golf and pitch and putt throughout my exam year. While all around me were stressed at the thought of sitting their first State exams, I got daily respite from all of it through physical exercise. I wasn't in tune with my mental health; in fact, I didn't know what the term 'mental health' really meant at this time. But I had made the association that physical exercise had a positive effect on my being as a whole, mind included.

My classmates were glad when the exams were all over, as was I. The day we finished, my classmates went one way and I went another. While most went in search of any amount of alcohol they could get their hands on ahead of house parties that night, I made my way to the GAA club to practise my frees. Nobody questioned why I wasn't joining them – by then, they knew none of that appealed to me.

In that summer of third year, the inter-county scene was getting slightly more serious. We were training twice a week in preparation for the Gerry Reilly Tournament – an under-sixteens tournament for teams from all around Leinster. A few of my teammates and I had aspirations to play Dublin minor football the following January, and the tournament was a good showcase to get you recognised.

Football wasn't the only thing I was representing Dublin in that summer. I was selected as part of a team of seven who represented Dublin in the Leinster and All-Ireland pitch and putt championships. We were successful in the initial stages and were crowned Leinster champions, but fell at the final hurdle, coming runners up in the All-Ireland to a very good Cork outfit. The football finished with us failing to reach the final of the Gerry Reilly Tournament, but I was hoping bigger things were just around the corner.

I entered fourth year knowing that it was time to make a decision: Would I choose Gaelic or soccer? I made my decision in December – I would go with Gaelic. I was selected to represent the Dublin minor footballers in January – my first year playing minor football for Dublin. Here I met a man who has been so pivotal in where I am today – Dessie Farrell, who was my Dublin minor manager for two years and my manager for three years at U21 level.

So, in January, we embarked on a journey that we hoped would bring us to the All-Ireland final in September. The perception people had of me, as the guy living an idyllic life, was further enhanced, particularly in school. When people asked me what I was up to, and I replied that I was training or playing a match for Dublin, it seemed to create an air of invincibility around me. Once the term 'Dublin footballer' was mentioned, people looked at and treated me differently. I never thought of myself as different; I just felt that I had an opportunity to do what I loved at the highest level.

The team's preparations began with the League, which ran until the start of April. We reached the League final, where we faced Longford, eventually coming out as eight-point winners. It was nice to pick up some silverware this early on in the campaign, but Dessie, as all great managers do, made us quickly put that to the back of our minds. We switched our focus to the next job at hand – the Leinster Championship.

We had navigated our way to the Leinster final by mid-July, overcoming Westmeath, Longford and Kildare in the process. In order to secure the Leinster Championship, we had to beat Meath in the final. A lacklustre display in the first half didn't leave much between us coming into the break. However, we were able to really turn on the style in the second half, and we ran out ten-point winners in the end; job done.

The momentum we had built throughout the Leinster Championship had us in prime condition going into the All-Ireland series. The goal that we had set ourselves way back in January – to reach the All-Ireland final – came to fruition, as we defeated Cork and Galway in the quarter- and semi-finals respectively. Unfortunately, we lost the All-Ireland final against Tipperary to a last-minute goal.

It was a bitter pill to swallow. For some, it was the end of the road at minor grade, but luckily for me and a number of others, we would have another chance the following year to win the Championship. However, little did I know about the challenges I was about to face.

CHAPTER 3

THE DARK DAYS

If I knew then what I know now, would things have been different? Would I have the same perspective on life? Would my life be better overall? These are questions I ask myself when I look back to January 2012, to the middle of fifth year, which marked the beginning of my depression. I was unaware then of the term 'depression', or 'mental health' for that matter. I thought the ebbing and flowing of my mood was due to hormonal changes in my body.

I had one purpose that year: to play a pivotal role in winning the minor All Ireland in September. The hurt from the previous year was still very raw. As a unit, we had lost the All Ireland. But personally, I hadn't quite reached the heights that were expected of me, and that I expected from myself. This really didn't sit well with me. Apart from a few brief appearances, I had essentially been a passenger for the entire year. This year, I had a point to prove. Nothing else mattered aside from football.

I remember my Mam saying, 'You've got to broaden your horizons. Open up your mind and see what life has to offer outside of football.' I would take no notice of such comments; I really couldn't see what she was getting at. I had tunnel vision. I was thinking about football from when my alarm went off for school in the morning right up until I lay my head to rest at night. That to me was normal.

What didn't seem normal were the periods of low mood I began to feel. They were very sporadic to start with, but there was one particular day in January that, when I think back, was perhaps the start of 'the dark days' for me.

It was mid-week, and I had a school football match to look forward to. The alarm woke me at 8am. Time to get up, but I had a strange feeling, like there was a weight on my shoulders. At first, I put it down to lack of sleep. However, after having a shower and breakfast, the feeling didn't subside. On my ten-minute walk to school, my emotions seemed to be going round and round on a conveyor belt. I was happy, sad, fearful – all of these emotions were rolling around in my head, and I didn't know how to make sense of them.

I arrived at the front gate of the school and was greeted by some friends. I felt engulfed by a heightened sense of awareness. I pushed down the emotions that were running through my mind, and adopted the mask that would become all too familiar over the next two years of my life.

The school day began. Being distracted by the classes that were in session and the short walks between those classes, there was little time for me to be in my own head. The team and I were due to meet after fourth period at the school car park, where the bus was to depart from for the match. I made my way into the toilet before heading up to the car park, and all of a sudden, I felt very low again.

A sense of panic gripped me – I couldn't be like this in front of the team, I thought. Of all the days to feel like this! Here I was, getting off school early to do what I loved best – to play football. I couldn't make sense of what was going on.

I made my way out of the toilet, still in a state of panic over how I was feeling, and walked to the car park. The team were packing their bags onto the bus and, much like that morning, the mask was placed on again – everything was 'fine' in my world. I took my customary seat, at the back left of the bus. I had very few superstitions leading up to a game, but this was where I had sat since the beginning of second year.

The bus took off, and we were on our way to the game. The noise level immediately rose, with different conversations going on throughout the length of the bus. I wouldn't be the loudest out of any group, though I would certainly usually have my say during the course of a conversation. But now a conversation had begun in my head, trying to make sense of what was going on for me, why I was feeling down.

I came in and out of the conversation in my head and the conversations going on in the bus. It was as if I had a set of noise-cancelling headphones, which I was putting on and taking off every few minutes. When I came back into the conversation on the bus, I feared was that one of my team-mates would ask why I was acting so weird. Thankfully though, this didn't happen.

I got out onto the pitch, and all my worries were whisked away. When the final whistle blew, and we went back onto the bus, the journey home was full of chat and laughter about the game. I was on a high, engrossed in the conversation going on around me – a stark contrast to the person who had sat on the bus a couple of hours earlier.

At home, settled in for an evening of television, I reflected on what had happened to me that day. I decided that there was nothing to worry about, and came to two very simple conclusions – number one, that it was just hormonal changes going on in my body; and number two, that I immediately felt better after playing the match. The latter would become a real crutch, something I would rely upon as my medication for the next few years.

Inter-county football was beginning to ramp up again. The Minor League was about to begin. I had learnt from the previous year that it was important to put my hand up early on in the League if I had any aspiration to get a starting place come Championship time in late April. I managed to get through the pre-season unscathed, and was in good shape coming into the start of the league.

It started off well, both for me and for the team as a collective. I was given the number nine shirt for the first couple of games, and we came out victorious in each. Every last ounce of my being that I had given in the pre-season seemed to be paying off. The League went according to plan, and we reached the final, which would be at the start of April, versus age-old rivals Meath.

For the majority of the League campaign, my mental health was relatively unaffected. However, two days before the League final, we had our last training session before the game. The team was due to be announced on that evening too. I arrived to training in Parnell Park confident that I would be given the number nine jersey again, but there was still a hint of doubt bubbling in my mind – 'What if?' I kept thinking to myself.

Training finished and, after showering and eating our post-session meal, the team meeting took place. There was great excitement, given that the League had gone so well, though there was some apprehension among the group too, as we were aware that many positions weren't nailed down by any means.

Dessie began to announce the team. I went to a place in my head far from the room that I was sitting in, only to rejoin the room as he approached his selection for the midfielders – 'Lining out in midfield will be Scooby and Shane Carthy ...' A huge sigh of relief escaped from me as I sank down into my chair. I could relax now, I was in.

The meeting went on for another hour or so. Dessie's meetings were notoriously long. Every little detail was driven home; no stone was left unturned. You left those meetings knowing that you would have no excuse come match day to say, 'I wasn't prepared for them to do this.' As the meeting drew to a close, I peered around the room. There were a lot of happy and relieved faces on those who had been given a starting place. Heading down the stairs, the group were in a jovial mood, looking forward to the task we were facing in two days' time.

I went out to the car park, where my Dad was waiting, leaning against the bonnet of his car. We made eye contact from about twenty metres away, and he gave me that questioning look, as if to say 'Are you in?' I briefly smiled to confirm that I was. I put my bag into the boot and sat into the car. My dad patted me on the head. 'Congratulations, son,' he said, and I could see the pride gleaming in his eyes.

On our short journey home, my Dad asked me the usual questions – who got in to the starting line-up, and who didn't? What sort of Meath team would be chosen? All the while, I was searching for the happiness that my dad was so clearly feeling for me. I couldn't search for too long, as the next question was being fired at me as soon as one was answered. My dad was unaware that I was completely zoned out for most of the journey home, trying to figure out why I wasn't overjoyed that I had been selected.

We arrived home, and I dropped my bag in the hall and made my way up to my room. It was getting late and I had school the following day. As I lay down in bed, I tried to convince myself that I was happy about the news

I had just received, but I just wasn't. I tossed and turned, asking myself, 'Why? Why am I feeling this way?' I eventually nodded off, no closer to an answer.

The next morning, I woke at 8am. I rose from the bed and cautiously walked into the bathroom. Everything seemed to be in slow motion. I was scanning through my mind and body to see if any of the emotions from the previous night had carried over to this morning. It was a strange feeling, as if I was tiptoeing through motion sensors, trying not to set them off. Once I got the all-clear that I felt 'normal' again in my head, I let out a sigh of relief.

We overcame Meath the following day in their own back yard. The team were brimming with confidence now, facing into the Championship. The first round was at the end of April, and we would face Carlow. The atmosphere was electric in the weeks leading up to the opening round. I had managed to perform well enough in the League final to warrant a starting place against Carlow.

Around school, particularly on Fridays, my classmates and friends would often slag me about my weekend plans. My weekends probably weren't like the majority of seventeen-year-olds. While the others discussed what fake ID they were going to use to get into a nightclub on Saturday night, I was thinking about training on Saturday morning, or what coach I needed to ask to get a bag of footballs to practise my free kicks on Sunday.

Although we always had a laugh and a joke about my weird lifestyle, I could feel that there was an underlying respect for the sacrifice and hard work I put in, week in, week out. I was, from a young age, placed up on a kind of pedestal, cast into the limelight, the untouchable figure around my school and area. I was never quite comfortable being this person, but because of my success in the sporting world, I found myself there nonetheless.

I coped with it all fine up until this juncture in my life, but the 'hormonal changes' now going on in my body wouldn't seem to leave me in peace. I didn't want to talk about it to anyone – to friends, family, coaches, anyone. I believed that I had a certain persona to live up to. The only thing I did know was that exercise worked for me. It got me feeling good about myself again when I did have those bad days. It was my crutch, my medication, and I relied upon it.

It was Friday, two days out from the first round of the Championship. I went to school as normal. I was sitting in English class, the last class before lunch break. Through the window I could see the training pitch, where we were due to train on our lunch break. I started feeling the dark cloud come over me again, the internal conversations beginning. I asked to go to the toilet so that I could try to figure this out alone. I locked myself in one of the cubicles, placed my hands on my head and began to ask myself the all-too-familiar question at this stage: 'Why?' I stood for a few minutes, convincing myself that I had nothing in my life that should make me feel this way – I had friends, family, a sporting career that was going well. 'I shouldn't be feeling this way' I kept saying. I started to feel tears building up, and this put me on high alert. 'If I start crying now, it'll be obvious when I go back into class,' I thought.

I reasoned that if I was back in class, with distractions and people around me, I'd have less time to think and I would most certainly hold back the tears in front of everyone. So I got out of the cubicle and made my way back to class. I sat myself down and tried to engage in as much class discussion as possible in order to drown out my internal conversations.

The bell rang at the end of class. My teammates and I went out onto the training pitch and into the school's pink dressing rooms to get changed.

I wasn't actually taking part in the session – I had Dublin training that evening and the match was also two days out. However, training or not, we were expected to be there. For the next forty minutes, the 'injured' lads and I watched on from the sidelines as the team trained.

As training came to a close, our manager, Mr O'Ceara, brought us in for a team huddle. He ended with, 'Best of luck to Shane Carthy this weekend, representing Dublin. The commitment and sacrifice you've shown to make it to here have to be acknowledged and admired. We're all very proud of you, as a school and also as a team.' There was a ripple of applause, along with a bit of good-natured jeering from some of the lads.

On my way back to class, the internal dialogue started yet again. That small gesture of good will from Mr O'Ceara, one that would make anyone feel good about themselves, did the opposite for me. In fact, it did two things: It made me ask, why can't I find the happiness that so many other people are clearly feeling for me? And it reinforced need to keep hiding away the fact that I was deeply unhappy, for fear of people either laughing at me or thinking I was lying.

I pushed down my feelings as I walked into the first class after lunch. I was almost in a state of paranoia, fearing that someone would spot something odd going on with me. I felt terror if anyone looked at me for a prolonged period of time. And along with this was a sad, down feeling, because I was feeling this way. My conveyor belt of emotions was in overdrive, and I had no way to stop it.

There were brief moments of respite when I was engrossed in school work, so I tried to focus on that for the remainder of the school day. As classes were coming to an end, I had one thing in my mind – home! Leaving school, I was wished good luck by lots of my fellow pupils. I couldn't appreciate or enjoy their good will, as all I wanted to do was escape.

I walked briskly home and placed my schoolbag in the hall. I called out, 'Anyone home?' Silence. I went up to my room, closed the door and sat down on my bed, head in hands. My mam generally arrived home around the same time as me, so I knew I didn't have long before I had to straighten up and put on that mask. For the time I was alone though, that conveyor belt was on overdrive. I felt tears building up, as they had earlier on that day. A few tears trickled down my cheek before I stood up abruptly and convinced myself to snap out of it. 'I can't cry, I can't,' I kept telling myself.

I changed out of my uniform and got my training gear ready for the session in a couple of hours. While I was doing this, my Mam arrived home. I went down to the kitchen where she was, and she asked me how my day was. Just like that, the mask went on. I quickly answered, 'Fine,' and escaped into the sitting room. Little did she know that my day was far from 'fine'. My whole being was far from 'fine'.

The wait for training made me anxious. I sat on the couch with the television on, in a daze. As I got in the car for training, the cloud in my head began to clear. The closer we got to the training ground, the clearer it was. I went out onto the training pitch, and the 'medication' I needed was right there, in the shape of a size five O'Neill's and an open field. Going home that evening, I found myself in a much better headspace.

We defeated Carlow a few days later, which meant we could look forward to a quarter-final meeting with Longford in a few weeks' time. It was a nice feeling, going into school on Monday morning and getting recognised by students and teachers alike for the past weekend's success. In fact, I felt good about myself for the entire week. My head was held a bitter higher, shoulders pushed back and a confidence in my stride.

The following week, while preparing for the Longford game, which was only five days away now, my boots ripped in training. I had to part ways with a pair of boots that had served me well, but the excitement of shopping for a new pair of boots trumped the disappointment. I had a half day the next day, as we did every Wednesday, so I said I'd make the short journey to Pavillions shopping centre to pick up a new pair. I was driving on a provisional license, and every so often my parents would give me the freedom to make short trips on my own in the car.

I was excited to be driving myself to Pavillions to pick up a new pair of boots, on a lovely, sunny day. As I approached the underground car park, my excitement dwindled somewhat. As I went from the sun to the darkness of the underground car park, it was as though my mind followed suit. A dark cloud surrounded my thoughts, and I was quickly feeling low yet again. I parked the car up, turned off the engine and sat, trying to compose myself.

A million thoughts rushed through my head and, not for the first time, I didn't know what to do. The silence in the car didn't help. I turned on the radio to try to distract my mind. That didn't work. I was in a trance. Every so often I would come out of this state and hear the sound of the radio, but only for short moments. A lot of the time, my mind was just blank. I sat, slumped, just stuck in this low mood. It was paralysing.

When I eventually picked my head up and peered at the clock, thirty minutes had passed. On my way out the door, my dad had said, 'Don't go anywhere except the shopping centre. You're lucky enough we're letting you out to drive on your own, and we'll know if you've been elsewhere.' This began to ring in my head. Normally, it wouldn't have been a big deal. However, what was going on in my head wasn't normal. The last thing I was going to do was to tell my Dad the truth as to why I was late home. I just couldn't face up to it. I was scared and embarrassed, and I felt trapped.

I got out of the car, put up the invisible mask and went into the shop. I still wasn't feeling quite right. It felt like it took an age for the shop assistant to fetch my tried and trusted Copa Mundial boots from the storeroom, but eventually I got them.

Rushing back to the car, my head was in a whirl. As I steered out of the car park, I thought of a hundred and one excuses I could give to my dad, should he ask why I was slightly late coming home. My mind was going back and forth between thinking of excuses and asking myself, 'Will this ever get better?' I never considered at this stage, even for a brief moment, telling someone how I was feeling. Repressing it all and making excuses for how I was feeling sat better with me.

My heart was racing as I approached the house. I was just hoping that I wouldn't have to make up an excuse, that nobody would notice that there was something not quite right with me. My dad's car wasn't in the drive. There was still the possibility that my mam was there though. I pulled into the drive and tentatively got out of the car. I was shaking as I put the key in the door.

I opened the door and let out a rather nervous 'hello'. No reply. I felt a huge weight slide off my shoulders. I went into the kitchen and made a cup of coffee. I didn't sit there for long though – I knew I would start ruminating again. I needed to get out of the house and do something. I decided to break in my new boots and practise free kicks up in the local GAA club.

On my way from my house to the club, a dull, dreary feeling was still hanging over me. However, once I began running around and kicking the ball, it was as though all my worries just drifted away. The person returning to the house after an hour up in the club was a stark contrast to the one who had walked in from the shopping centre only a few hours previously.

That evening, I sat in my room, worrying about where my mind was taking me. It was happening more and more now. I wasn't in control of my emotions, and I didn't know how much worse it was going to get. How long could I keep up the facade that everything in my life was going fine, when in reality it wasn't? One thing I did know though – exercise was my escape. I would put all my trust in this, in the hope that things would get better.

The school week came to an end, and now there was only one thing that mattered – the Leinster quarter-final versus Longford. I kept my place from the previous match, and I was raring to go. Training was good medication to get me through this difficult patch, but matches were the golden panacea for me. On match day, it was impossible to be concerned about anything else in life.

Internally, I would visualise everything to do with the lead up to the match and the match itself, even before anything had happened. This day was no different. I woke up and had my usual match-day breakfast – a bowl of porridge with honey and natural yoghurt mixed in, a cup of orange juice and a coffee. For the next couple of hours, I sat watching television. Then it was time to pack my gear bag. Many players pack everything the night before, but I do it differently. I haven't got many superstitions leading up to a game, but I suppose packing my bag on the day of a match is one of them.

Now my pre-match meal of chicken and pasta, a staple for many sports people, was awaiting me. When that was inhaled in record time, it was time to go and do what I loved best, to play football. Nothing was out of the ordinary as we arrived at Parnell Park. Players were doing their thing in preparation for the match – some sitting listening to music, others getting taped up by the physio, some having a chat. The time came to go out and compete for a place in the Leinster semi-final. There were no second chances; everything was on the line.

After a tense affair, we managed to come out as victors. I was delighted personally too, having played an important role throughout and having chipped in with a few points. I was in good spirits coming home, and that feeling continued throughout the evening, sitting at home with my family. However, when I woke the following morning, the dreaded dark cloud had engulfed my mind once more. I reached over to turn off the alarm and sat up in bed, and took a few moments to check in with myself. I felt terrible, and the situation was compounded by the fact that I felt bad for feeling bad.

I could hear murmurs from my parents and sister down in the kitchen. I decided I would have a shower and try to compose myself before going downstairs. My mind was racing again. Standing in the shower with my head down and shoulders hunched, I felt exhausted already, worrying about having to put on a show in front of everyone for the day. For the next few hours at least, I would have to put on that mask, as I had to go to the GAA club and support my team, who were playing a League match that morning. I knew I'd have kids and adults alike coming up to me to congratulate me on the previous day's victory over Longford.

In the kitchen, I told my parents I was going to the GAA club straight away, to help out with preparing the jerseys, cones and balls for the match. This wasn't actually the case. It was an hour until throw-in, and no one was expecting me there beforehand. Instead, I went to the car park at the local beach. I knew it wouldn't be too busy, as the weather was pretty overcast.

I was going against what I knew worked for me when I needed to distract my mind, which was keeping active. I thought, by some divine miracle, if I took some time to myself I could figure out what was going on inside me. This was a losing battle, because when I asked myself, 'Okay, what is making me feel this way?' I simply had no response. Instead, negative feelings raced through my body, and I was like a rabbit in headlights.

If I hadn't thought it before, I knew now that whatever was going on for me, it was taking control of my life. The word 'depression' never came into my mind, simply because I had never heard that word.

I was surprised to see people coming into the car park and onto the beach, on such a grey day. I began to feel uneasy – the cloud over my mind hadn't subsided, and I was fearful that someone would come by who knew me and start asking questions as to why I was there.

I drove out of the car park, and up to the GAA club. My body was trembling as I pulled up. It was a busy morning at the club, with matches and training going on across all five pitches. I glanced at myself in the mirror to make sure there wasn't anything externally wrong with me, in fear that it would raise a red flag for someone. I looked okay. I wasn't quite like that internally though – inside I was screaming for help.

Walking over to the dressing room where management and players were, I remember saying to myself, 'Don't let yourself down.' It was as though there were two people inside me. One was small in stature, frail and in desperate need of help, while the other was all-conquering and decisive. This stronger character was the one winning over my mind.

Upon reaching the dressing room, I drew a deep breath, put on my invisible mask and began being the person that I thought everyone expected to see. As soon as I engaged in conversation with one of my teammates, this act I was putting on started to slot into place. We talked about the match the day before, about school finishing up and a summer of football to look forward to, with even a chance to play in Croke Park again. Sure, what could go wrong in my life? I was the laughing, energetic, 'not a care in the world' type of guy they wanted me to be.

Standing at the side of the pitch, talking to parents and players during the game, nothing seemed out of place. To put the icing on the cake, when the match ended and I was walking back to the car, a few club juvenile players approached me and asked for a picture. I, of course, duly obliged. I smiled and joked with them momentarily, then headed off to my car. On the way home, I actually didn't feel so bad anymore. It seemed like I had nearly convinced myself that I was the person everyone had seen up at the club. I spent the rest of my afternoon with friends.

At home that evening, I noticed how tired I was. I wasn't physically tired, but I was mentally exhausted. I knew straight away it was from the acting performance I had put on earlier in the day. What worried me was that this was just one day. How much more of this would I have to do before things get better? Little did I know what was to come.

The end of the school year was in sight. Inter-county football would take a back seat for a couple of weeks, to make way for the Leaving Certificate. Thankfully, all I had to worry about was my fifth year summer exams. I was never the most studious, but I always did relatively okay come exam time. My worry this time though wasn't the exams themselves, but whether my mind would let me sit still and take in information. One thing had become very clear to me – sitting still, having time to ruminate, took my mind to very dark places.

As I sat down to study, just two weeks before the exams, I was worried. The first subject to tackle was Maths, as this would be my first exam. I handled the Maths book as if it were an explosive. I opened the book in slow motion, intending to attempt a few sample questions that might come up in the exam. Putting pen to paper, every so often I would pause, to check that everything was okay. This was the crippling effect the depression I was going through was having on my everyday life. The past five months had been like nothing I had experienced before.

As my studies went on, I noticed I got into more of a flow, and I started to worry less about negative thoughts that might enter my mind. When I closed the book and put my pen down, I leaned back in my chair and pondered for a moment. A smile spread across my face. The worry and doubt I had felt beforehand was gone, and a calmness ran through my mind and body. I decided that, like physical activity, studying seemed to have a positive effect on me. Physical activity was an escape and a coping mechanism for me, but I didn't see studying in the same way. I simply saw that it could help me to keep up an appearance. I was bottling up all these emotions, and I didn't want anyone to spot any cracks in my character; not being able to study would have meant not getting the results I had in previous years, which would have waved a red flag to my teachers and parents. Questions would arise if I had poor results, and I would have had to make up excuses to explain them.

The following few weeks of study continued to have a therapeutic effect, right up until the first day of exams. There were a few days where I felt low in myself, but never for any length of time. The night before my first exam, I was doing a final bit of preparation and feeling quite good. My head was in a good place.

Waking up on the morning of the first exam, I was actually quite excited. I think this was mostly because if the exams were about to start, then the end wasn't too far away! I got everything I would need packed into my bag, and I headed out to school. The exams would take place in the PE hall, where two year groups would sit their exams, first years and fifth years. You could feel the energy in all the students as we waited for the doors to be opened. You could see the fear and worry in the first years' faces as they prepared to sit their first summer exam. Among my year, fifth year, there was a slightly more relaxed atmosphere, but still the odd worried face.

The doors eventually opened, and we all made our way in to find our seats with their assigned numbers. With the aid of the teachers, everyone found their seat and began to settle. This wasn't the first time I'd been in the PE hall with this many people. Two years previously, I had sat here doing my Junior Certificate, alongside Leaving Certificate students. However, I found myself in a daze, looking over my left and right shoulders at the sheer masses of people in the hall.

Attention was brought to the front of the hall, where the teachers notified us that the exam papers were about to be passed around. As the papers were passed out row by row, I began to narrow my focus on the job at hand. Just like the in previous couple of weeks, I could now solely focus on answering the questions that were in front of me.

The ninety-minute exam seemed to fly by, and I finished with about five or ten minutes to spare. Now my mind began to wander. I looked around at the crowd of pupils in the hall. 'What if the dark clouds come over my head again and I can't leave the exam hall?' I thought to myself. Then, 'What if I do get up? I'll have three hundred eyes burning into the back of my head'. I was thinking irrationally, but I couldn't snap out of it.

Just as the negative emotions began to snowball, time was up for the exam. The teachers began to collect the papers, and the usual chatter echoed around the hall. Thankfully, I was too distracted by conversation to be in my own head walking out. I found my friend Moe and we made our way back to my house for lunch. It was a godsend that he came home with me, because it meant I had less time to be brooding. At that time, I felt like the dark clouds could descend at any moment.

We had a couple of hours before we had to head back to school for our second exam of the day. We spent the time making some lunch and then sitting down to chat about anything and everything. I felt the clouds begin to dissipate as the conversation went on. I was learning the powerful effect that conversation could have on my mental state.

I relied upon this for the remainder of my exams. Some days I felt like I wanted to talk to someone in my family or a best friend. However, never once did I think about bringing up what was really going on for me. Instead, the conversation centred on sport, friends, family … all that normal stuff. It worked when my mind felt like it was taking over, but in reality, this was all masking over bigger problems that would come later down the line. Other days, when I didn't feel like talking but still needed to clear my head, I would go out and exercise.

Now, with the exams out of the way, I switched my attention to the next round of the Championship, a little over five weeks away. For the next couple of weeks, numbers were down at training, due to some people sitting the Leaving Certificate. Those of us who had no exams now had a chance to get ahead and get noticed. You could feel the energy and excitement in the group – hot summer days, grafting away at gruelling training sessions that we all knew would put us in good stead for five weeks' time. I loved every minute of it.

I had very little else going on in my life at that time, and I chose to have it that way. Everything revolved around football. My time away from training was spent thinking about training. If my friends planned something – say, a walk down the beach – and I thought it would have a negative effect on my performance on the pitch, I'd stay at home and rest up. My friends were used to me cancelling plans because of football. This also gave me the perfect excuse to cancel when I didn't feel so good mentally.

I recall one particular weekend when this was the case. We were three weeks out from the Championship semi-final. We had training on the Friday evening, the weekend off to enjoy with friends and family and training again on the Monday. I loved to get out and play golf when I could, and this was an ideal time to take advantage of the couple of days off. Earlier in the week I had contacted my friend Karl and organised a game of golf for the Saturday. I texted him after training on the Friday evening to reconfirm our plans.

Things very quickly changed on the Saturday morning though. I woke up with the summer sun fighting its way through my curtains. Internally, however, there were no rays of sun. Instead, the dreaded dark clouds were quickly assembling.

For anyone who hasn't experienced depression, it can be hard to relate to the 'dark clouds' that come over you. If I was talking about a broken leg or a broken heart, things would be different; it would be much easier to feel empathy and compassion for the person going through it. But these dark clouds feel as though someone with a remote control is constantly changing channel, flicking from one negative emotion to the next. It is like carrying a bag on your back weighing a tonne, and no matter how much you want to take it off, you can't. It's exhausting.

This was exactly how I felt upon waking this particular morning. The 'mental health toolbox' that might help me might as well have been located on a different planet. The last thing I felt able to do was to get up and get active, or even talk to someone. I knew I needed to stop the spiral, but the voice inside my head simply wouldn't let me. Instead, I lay there ruminating, letting the tap of negative emotion fill my body. I tried to think of a happy moment or something funny that had happened recently, but I wasn't able to attach a positive emotion to anything.

I eventually emerged from my bed, and even that felt like a huge effort. I headed in to the shower, attempting to re-gather my thoughts and find a way out of this paralysis. I would have to find an excuse for why I couldn't play golf that afternoon. My mind raced through every excuse possible. I wrote a text message saying that I had an inter-county friendly instead of training on Monday, and therefore I couldn't go out in the baking sun for four to five hours, expending all my energy so close to a game. Ashamed at how I was feeling and the lies I was telling, I pressed 'send'. I threw my phone on the bed and sat down with my head in my hands. Shame, anger, guilt and sadness all flooded over me.

Outside my window, I could hear a couple of local kids screaming and laughing, playing football out in the back field. I would have done anything to feel like they did in that moment. For about six months now, I had held everything back and got through it somehow. But at that moment, I felt exhausted. The tears that I'd been holding back for a long, long time now began to flow, and I did nothing to stop them. I was telling myself to stop crying, but the tap kept flowing. After about five minutes and with a river of tears beneath me, I gathered myself together somewhat.

When my tears had dried and I let out a huge exhale, I felt slightly better.

I stayed in my room for another while before coming downstairs to my family, to wait for the redness in my eyes to subside. As I went into the kitchen, my dad asked what time I was leaving to play golf. I repeated the excuse that I had a match on Monday, so I needed to rest up. I was slightly nervous to see whether or not he would buy the lie I was telling him. He did.

I went into the sitting room, exhausted. All this was becoming too much. A text came through from Karl, and my heart rate increased ever so slightly. 'No problem ...' it read. I let out a huge sigh of relief and sank a little deeper into the couch.

After a while of staring blankly at the television, I started to regret cancelling the day's plans. Now I wanted to get out of the house and occupy my mind. I shouted in to my dad, and asked him if he wanted to go up to the GAA club with me to practise free kicks ahead of the 'game' on Monday. 'Yes,' he said. My mood instantly lifted. I was absolutely perplexed by how my mind was working, going from feeling desperately low one minute to happy and excited the next.

Dad and I headed up to the GAA club and began my usual routine of kicking seventy-five to one hundred balls. I strived for excellence in absolutely everything I did on the football field. Once I set down the ball and began my rigid routine, I was engrossed. It was a welcome break from the inner turmoil I was experiencing.

My kicking was going well and my mood continued to lift. Retrieving the twelve footballs we had each time gave my dad and I time to talk. We chatted away about the upcoming semi-final in three weeks' time. I knew that small things like going to the GAA club to help me with my free kicks meant the world to him. It was etched on his face. In years gone by, he had helped out with coaching at the club.

As I went on with my free kicks, I had momentary thoughts of telling my dad that I was going through a difficult period. But I quickly chased these notions away.

I kicked my final ball, which split the posts, to end a very good day's kicking. It was like taking my last bit of medicine to help me get through the day, and a smile broke out from ear to ear with sheer delight at how I was feeling physically. Mentally, with those post-exercise endorphins coursing through my body, I was feeling good too.

'That's the best I've seen you strike the ball in a very long time,' said my dad. When you're at such a low point in your life, comments like this mean the world. Heading home in the car, I felt ten feet tall.

The summer holidays were in full swing, and I had a lot of time on my hands, especially during the day. I had learned that keeping busy meant I would spend less time thinking negative thoughts, so I decided to look for part-time work to fill the void. I sent out a number of CVs and began to look around. One evening, my friend Glenn told me that he was about to start work with his mam in the school that she was principal of. By a stroke of luck, she was looking for another worker to help out in a summer camp being held over the next three weeks. Glenn asked his mam if I could come and work for her at the summer camp and, without a moment's hesitation, she answered, 'Yes, of course.'

Things were looking up. Two weeks out from a semi-final against Kildare, and I now had a part-time job to keep me busy during the day. I constantly reaffirmed that thought, telling myself that the past five months were now behind me and I could now look forward to all these good things in my life.

Monday morning came, the first day of the summer camp. I woke up extra early, eager to get my day going and my mind occupied. Glenn and his mother, Grainne, picked me up down the road and we made our way to St Malachy's boys' national school. Setting up the school hall, I tried my best to get around to everyone and introduce myself. The children began arriving, and Glenn and I were assigned a group together. I was a little nervous at first, but I quickly got the hang of things and felt comfortable. The whole day went by without any issues – in fact, it was very enjoyable.

I would never be one to announce myself as 'Shane Carthy, Dublin footballer'; it was always simply 'Shane Carthy'. But of course, somewhere during the day Glenn happened to mention that I played football for Dublin, and this immediately sparked interest, not only among the children, but among the adults working there too. I imagine my reaction would have been similar when I was a youngster. When the tag 'Dublin footballer' was attached to the end of your name, people instantly treated you differently. I always got the sense, even if they weren't saying it out loud, that they were certainly saying to themselves internally, 'You have a great life, playing for Dublin, in Croke Park with thousands of fans watching on – an idyllic life.' I can only speak for myself, but I felt a certain responsibility to live up to that expectation, that perception others had of me. I had no reason to feel anything but happy in my life – what could possibly go wrong for a seventeen-year-old, playing for Dublin, with a loving family and friends?

Little did anyone know the effect that Glenn's harmless and innocuous comment would have on me. For the rest of that day, the children at the summer camp were coming up to me, asking what it was like to play for Dublin. I could see their ears perk up, hungrily consuming every last word I said to them. The workers also asked me all sorts of questions, saying things like, 'It must be so great,' and, 'That's not a bad life you have.'

When I got home later that day, I couldn't get people's reactions and comments out of my head. I sat up in my room and began ruminating once more. I blamed myself for feeling down the past five months, when anyone else would have loved to be in my shoes. 'Why am I feeling this way? What have I to be sad about? These people are right, I do have a great life,' I told myself. I was confused and upset, and scared to tell anyone I was feeling this way. All the fun and excitement of working in the summer camp came crumbling down.

I didn't spend long sitting in my room, because I knew my parents and sister would be home shortly, meaning it was time to put up that poker face. My daily dose of 'medication', in the shape of a gym session, wasn't too far away, so I got prepared for that. I began enumerating short-term things that I had to look forward to. In ten days' time, I had the Leinster semi-final. I had the gym and pitch sessions leading up to it, and then the match itself. If I found myself feeling down, the next gym or pitch session was never too far away and I could focus in on that.

However, the next ten days were increasingly difficult working in the school. There were moments when I would pretend I needed to go to the toilet when in reality I had to regain my composure because I felt the mask breaking. At home, I was lying about how work was going.

I was so relieved when the end of the week came. The constant effort of putting on this act was exhausting. Not for one second did I think about throwing in the towel though, or telling anyone how I was feeling. The end of my short-term target was in sight. Having busied myself over the weekend with training, socialising and anything else that could keep my mind occupied, I was ready for one final push toward the match that Wednesday. In a way, I was doing the right thing by putting plans in place to occupy my mind for brief spells, but I was ignoring the elephant in the room. Depression makes you susceptible to irrational thinking, and that's what was happening, though I was fully aware that my mind wasn't functioning the way it should be.

Monday came, two days out from the Leinster semi-final. When I walked through the gates of the school, the acting mode button had been switched on and I was ready for yet another audition. Like the previous week, I wasn't feeling one hundred percent in my head, but I put my best poker face on in front of the workers and children. The more the day went on, the more I kept blaming myself for feeling the way I did. Any other person would love to be in my shoes, I kept thinking. The ever-growing dark cloud that was engulfing my mind wouldn't let me see the positives in the life I was living. We would have training that evening, and that is where I switched my attention to any time I found myself drifting into a spiral of negative thoughts.

The work day eventually came to a close. I got home and began to pack my bag for training. The routine checklist – boots, gloves, shorts, socks and a training top – were all ticked off, and I was set to go. While everything else in my life seemed to be whittling away, these five items were keeping me afloat. Like any time I was in a difficult place, the only place in the world I wanted to be was on a football field. The inner demons were put on mute, for a couple of hours at least.

There was a certain amount of apprehension going in to hear the team announcement, but I was fairly confident of a starting position. My confidence was soon reaffirmed, with Dessie naming me to start alongside Scooby yet again. I headed home that evening on cloud nine. I wanted to press a fast forward button on my life, to get me to Wednesday evening's game.

Work flew by the following day. The dark clouds never came to visit, and I was so thankful for that. I spent time that evening with my two best friends, Karl and Moe. It was comforting that I didn't have to put on an act in front of them; we could just enjoy each other's company. I headed home at a reasonable hour to rest up for the game the following day.

I was grateful to have match day off work. I went through my usual routine of breakfast, chill-out time and packing my gear bag. I had lots of time on my hands – we weren't due to meet until 4pm, as the match was at 7pm. This meant I had more time to be in my own head.

Usually I would've got out of the house to distract myself with some form of physical activity. However, this wasn't an option with the game pending. I didn't even consider a walk, because I was paranoid about expending unnecessary energy prior to the game. I had a slight concern hovering over my head. It had been a while since my last bus journey with a team, and that one didn't go too smoothly. Even though I was in good spirits, I knew this probably wouldn't last the whole day. I started to think about things that could keep me distracted on the bus, things that wouldn't draw too much attention to me at the same time. Many ideas popped into my head, but the most obvious and simple one was music. Apart from the inevitable chatter that goes on in a team bus, there are always those mute players that stick the headphones on and prepare for the match that way.

I began to gather up songs on my phone that reminded me of a happy time or place with friends and family, and I put them into a playlist. The loud music ringing in my ears, summoning positive memories from the past, would be the perfect cure for any negative feelings that might come into my head. I had all genres in my playlist, anything and everything that would conjure up a happy moment in time for me – Stevie Wonder, Elton John, Jay-Z, Eminem, Coldplay, all sorts of stuff.

Now it was time to get changed into my Dublin tracksuit and meet up with the team. I was in good spirits arriving at the hotel for the pre-match meal. The atmosphere was quite relaxed. Our meal selection generally consisted of rice, pasta, chicken, beef, vegetables, salad, fruit, juice, tea and coffee. I always cast an eye over what others consumed pre-match. For some it would be two or three plates of food, while others would have one small serving.

When the meal was consumed, I grabbed a cup of coffee and found a quiet spot. I put my headphones on and had one last look over my notes on the individual I would be facing. Other players would be getting strapped by the physiotherapist, or sitting around chatting.

Before the bus departed for Kildare, Dessie gathered us in for a short pre-match brief. He stood at the front of the room with the tactics board, delivering a few key messages on the opposition and then focusing in on us and our game plan. Then we all boarded the bus and headed off for Kildare.

Some players were very particular in where they sat on the bus, so there was an unwritten rule that you didn't sit in their seat. I was never too superstitious, but my seat was the second seat in on the very back right, and that's where I sat for the rest of the campaign. Sitting to the left of me was our corner back, Ross McGowan, and directly in front of him was our full back and captain, David Byrne.

After a short chat, everyone settled into the journey. I stuck in my headphones and went away to my own world in my head. As we got closer to the ground, I visualised how I would like to play in the game. This was something that many coaches encouraged us as players to do. You would often hear them say, 'start thinking about the game now.' I was a firm believer in it, and I found it had a positive impact on my game the majority of the time. Unknown to me at the time, I would rely heavily upon the power of visualisation and role play later down the line, in a different context.

We reached the ground, and made our way into the dressing room. Now we had fifteen minutes of our own time. Like many players, I liked to go out and have a walk around the pitch before heading back inside to get ready for the game. I found comfort in that routine.

As Dessie came in to have a last word, you could sense a few nerves among the group. At this stage of the Championship, it was do or die. You lose, your Championship is finished. For many, it was their first taste of football at this level, so the nerves were understandable. We were also going out to face a very good Kildare side, in their own backyard. Dessie reminded us of the sacrifices we had all made to be there, and then outlined the key points of how we would impose our game plan. Then we made our way out onto the pitch to shape our destiny for the summer.

St Conleth's Park is a small ground, which makes for a hostile atmosphere. As the warm ups came to a close and we lined up for the national anthem, a buzz ringing around the ground, we were all thinking 'this is it'. The game began and, as expected, it was a tight and tense affair. For much of the first half, both teams traded score for score, leaving it level coming into the half time break.

We entered the dressing room and split off into backs and forwards for a debrief. We all felt there was much more in us and that the game was there for the taking. Dessie came in and echoed the same feeling. He said all the right things, ending with, 'Thirty minutes to decide where your season goes.'

Going out for the second half, the nerves that were hanging over us in the first half seemed to have dissipated. There was an air of confidence among the collective and it showed throughout the half. We ran out convincing winners in the end. Our reward would be a Leinster final versus Meath in Croke Park, in two and a half weeks' time.

It was an incredible feeling, walking off the pitch, being congratulated by so many adoring Dublin fans, both young and old. The adrenaline was pumping, and happy endorphins were running through my body.

There were fantastic celebrations in the dressing room afterwards. So many hours of work had been put in, both by management and players, to make it to this point. You could see the relief etched across many faces around the dressing room.

Everyone finished showering up and we began to emerge from the dressing room in dribs and drabs, to make our way to the bus. Waiting outside were parents and fans that still wanted to pass on their congratulations. I found my mam and dad, who were visibly proud. I told them I would travel home in the car with them – I wanted to get to bed early, as I had work in the morning. They asked, would I not like to go back on the bus and enjoy the celebrations with the lads on the journey home? But even though I was in a good headspace and very much enjoying the celebrations with the lads, there was still that voice on my shoulder reminding me of the threat of an incoming dark cloud. The last place I wanted to be was on that bus should a dark cloud appear over my head. If it did and I was in the car with just my mam and dad, it would be easier to handle.

The lads were creating unforgettable memories on the journey home that night, memories that a young aspiring footballer should have after a victory like that. But I was being robbed of these because of the stranglehold my mind had on me. At that moment, once I kept the dark clouds at bay, I was content. I was in such fear of them coming back I would do anything to help deter them.

Next, I was very much looking forward to the preparations for the upcoming Leinster final. Over the following few weeks, I lived a highly regimented lifestyle. If I wasn't working alongside Glenn in the school, I was never too far away from a football and a pitch. While my friends went out socialising, I preferred to sit in to rest for the next training session. I did meet up with my close friends Karl and Moe for coffee some days, or called over to watch television, but that was about it. Nothing mattered to me apart from football.

In my quiet, alone time around this period, my mind would wander off to a sunny Croke Park, which would get all sorts of senses tingling in my body. However, there were still days around this time that had me feeling down. Morning time was when I was most likely to have negative feelings. I had plenty to look forward to during these days, leading up to the Leinster final, but yet I still felt this way. I could never quite figure it out. These low moods were never so severe that I felt like hiding myself away though. I could go about my day, but it felt like I had a cap on how much joy I could bring into my life.

A week before the Leinster final, I finished up working in the summer camp with Glenn and his mother. This left a massive void in my mornings and afternoons. I knew that keeping active and occupying my mind kept the low moods at bay, so I started to jot down things that I enjoyed doing on a piece of paper. Each day, I would pick one or two things on the sheet to do so that I kept busy – going on a long drive to a café, with a playlist of my favourite songs to listen to on the way; a walk with friends; going to the driving range to hit a few golf balls; or an extra session in the gym.

None of these things was unusual for me to do, so no alarm bells were raised with my family or friends. There were mornings when it didn't work, when I didn't want to meet up with friends or go to cafés. However, the one constant that I could always rely on was football training. No matter how bad it got, training would always take me to a better place.

The Monday, Wednesday and Friday of that week were my 'bankers' as we prepared for the Leinster final that coming Sunday. I had a positive start to my week, putting into play my distraction techniques in addition to the training sessions. The mood amongst my teammates was at an all-time high as we looked forward to stepping out into Croke Park for the first time this year. For some players it was going to be their first time playing at the stadium. Others had had the experience of it the previous year. I had a brief twenty-minute cameo in the previous year's Leinster final, but this was set to be my first start there. Regardless of how many times you set foot onto that pitch, it's always a very special occasion.

My week was going well right up until the Friday. As was becoming the norm at this stage, I woke up in a funk with little to no understanding of why. My plan on this day was to meet up with Karl and Moe for some lunch, to kill a few hours before the final training session leading up to the game. First I made breakfast, prepared my training gear for that evening and looked at some clips of the opponents we would be facing that week-end. I was hoping to stay distracted, to derail my negative train of thought and focus on the match at the weekend. It was a battle between two streams of emotions, each trying to get the upper hand.

After only a few minutes of staring blankly into the computer screen, the negative side had won. I was quickly spiralling into negative emotion upon negative emotion. If the prospect of playing in Croke Park in two days' time couldn't make me happy, then what would? I thought. I shut down the computer, stood up and walked out of the room. I spent a few minutes pacing up and down the hall, condemning myself for the negative train of thought I found myself in.

Hanging around the house wasn't going to do me much good. I needed to get out, so I made my way out to Howth slightly ahead of time. We were meeting in the Dog House, a café right beside the picturesque Howth Harbour. I parked up and went for a stroll around the harbour. Hearing the waves crashing up against the wall, the wind at my back and the seagulls flying overhead was a welcome intrusion into the noise going on in my head. It cast me back to my younger years. When my mam and I were walking or visiting scenic places, she would say, 'Be present and appreciative of your surroundings.' As a naïve and hormonal teenager, I would always laugh when she said things like that. But I began to realise that simple things, like walking by the sea, can really help you to appreciate life and how beautiful things are.

I got a text from Karl to say himself and Moe were five minutes away. I turned back towards the café, relieved that I had regained a bit of composure in my thinking. Sitting down to lunch, inevitably conversation turned to the match, coming up in two days' time. Earlier that morning, I couldn't have looked forward to the match, or even discussed it. But now, I got that rush of blood, that excitement and anticipation back. Strange how something as simple as a walk and a chat can change your mood so dramatically.

After lunch, I headed home to get ready for training. No matter what mood I was in, I was always like a kid on Christmas waiting to get out on the field. This training session was no different. We just did a small bit of skills, working on set plays and then finishing off with some individual work. It was more about the meeting afterwards, where the finer details of the game would be covered. Dessie was always so meticulous in his preparations, which gave us players confidence, knowing that there wouldn't be any surprises on match day. These meetings could go on for over an hour though, and it is mentally challenging to tune in for that entire time.

There was never an issue with tuning in when the team announcement came around, however. By this stage of the Championship, you would have a good idea beforehand whether you'd be starting or not. Nevertheless, I was anxious until Dessie got down to naming midfield, 'Shane Carthy and Scooby'. After the final words from Dessie, we were left to our own devices until Sunday morning.

I was elated leaving the grounds of DCU. At home, my parents were waiting in anticipation to learn whether I was to start. They were of course delighted for me, particularly my dad. I think he placed a lot of his joy and happiness around what I was doing in my sporting life. I guess he saw how much it all meant to me and wanted me to succeed at it, like any father would.

It took me a while to get to sleep that night, with the excitement of the occasion coursing through my body. The following day I hadn't much planned. I spent much of it going from the sitting room to the kitchen every couple of hours, to make sure my nutrition was on point for the following day. In the evening, a few of my friends called over to the house. They didn't stay for long, as they were aware I needed a good night's rest. Of course, I spent a good portion of the night tossing and turning with the excitement of the game the following day.

Then it was match day. I was up before my 8am alarm, hardly able to contain myself with the prospect of a Leinster final before me. We weren't due to meet up until 11.15am, but I always liked to be up in good time. The week leading up to a big match like this can be mentally draining, because it's almost all you think about. The morning of the match is probably even worse.

I did my level best on this morning not to get too fixated about the match in my head. The house was busy, with my parents, sister Stephanie, sister Michelle and her boyfriend all around. I kept my mind occupied, talking all things non-football with them all. With the team meeting time fast approaching, I went upstairs and gathered up my gear.

My two teammates and good friends Stephen Cunningham – Scooby as he was known – and Conor Ryan were collecting me to give me a lift to DCU. I sat up front with Stephen at the wheel and Conor in the back. Scooby was of course in charge of the tunes. I was never the biggest fan of Scooby's choice of songs, but some particular songs were becoming an integral part of our journeys to training and indeed matches. Some of them would later find themselves in my playlist at a time I needed them the most.

After an entertaining twenty-minute car journey, we arrived at DCU's St Clare's sports campus. We would be there for about an hour before the team bus was due to bring us to Croke Park. We had our pre-match meal and then a pre-match brief, reinforcing our game plan and ensuring that everyone knew their individual job.

Dessie closed out the meeting, and we all gathered our bags and got onto the bus. Almost everyone sat in exactly the same seat they had sat in the last time, when we faced Kildare. With Ross sitting to the left of me and David in front, I stuck on my earphones and began to focus in on the game. As Croke Park got closer, the volume on the bus lowered and lowered. The first sight of the stadium made everything very real. The time was now. The big blue gates swung open to let the bus into the tunnel. We then drove underground towards our dressing room, on the Cusack

Stand side. Coming off the bus with television cameras in our faces was something we were used to from the previous year's few visits.

In the dressing room, our jerseys were hanging, all perfectly numbered. I placed my bag down where the number nine shirt was, feeling a brief moment of pride. We had twenty minutes before the pre-match preparations, and myself and the majority of the lads went out to walk the hallowed turf of Croke Park. It's an incredible feeling to step out in Croke Park at any time, but particularly on Leinster final day. It felt a little eerie, because the stadium was so empty and quiet. After a short walk on the pitch, we went back into the dressing room to get changed.

All our movement-based stuff was done in what is called the 'green room', right next to the dressing room. This is relatively small in size, probably about fifteen metres by ten metres. As if it wasn't going already, warming up in there really gets the adrenaline going. In such a tight and enclosed area, you can literally bounce off the energy coming from teammates.

Next, we went back to the dressing room to hear Dessie's last words before heading out onto the pitch for the final part of the warm up. Now, as we emerged from under the Cusack Stand, there was a crowd of about 20,000 people watching on. The warm up flew by, and then it was time to line up for the national anthem. 'Amhrán na bhFiann' being played was a special moment to savour, and then it was game time.

As usual, once I was immersed in the game, it was all I could think about. The first half was a pretty cagey affair, but we went in at the break with a slight advantage. We regrouped at half time, knowing that we were better than what we had shown individually and collectively in the first half. The commencement of the second half showed just that – we got off to a quick start, and eventually ran out comfortable winners.

When the final whistle blew, joy was evident across everyone's face – the first of the two trophies we were chasing that year had been secured. Our captain, David Byrne, went up the steps of the Hogan Stand to lift the Father Larry Murray Trophy, and we followed with the traditional lap of the pitch.

The celebrations continued in the dressing room afterwards. It felt as though the cap that was recently put on the amount of joy I could bring into my life was lifted. I loved every second of it. We eventually calmed down, showered up and made our way back onto the bus. Victory chants were heard the entire length of the bus all the way back to DCU. The plan was to head home, and then meet back up later in Na Fianna GAA club, where the celebrations would really begin.

Scooby dropped me home and I was greeted by my delighted parents in the hallway. As usual, my dad asked me a million and one questions about the game, and about my performance in particular. It was almost like a miniature milestone for him, as he had been part of my success since day one.

As the conversation finished, I got a few moments to myself in my room. The joy that I had felt earlier in the day now felt like it was being clouded over again. While I was getting ready to go out to Na Fianna, the internal dialogue in my head began to tell me not go out for drinks, for fear of my low mood coming back – I might have to put on an act in front of my teammates, and with drink on me too. I thought about it a bit longer and came to a decision: So as not to arouse any suspicion, I would go to Na Fianna, have one or two drinks and ask someone from my family to come and pick me up before my teammates headed on from the club. I wasn't a big drinker anyway, so I thought this wouldn't seem out of the ordinary.

I headed downstairs, where my family were all congregated around the kitchen table. The team was due to meet up at 8pm, so I asked my family whether one of them could collect me at 10pm from the club. Inevitably, I was asked, 'Why aren't you heading out for the whole night to celebrate?' 'I don't want to celebrate fully until we win the All Ireland,' I replied. My response was met with some laughter around the table. My sister said, 'Would you ever relax and enjoy yourself for one night?' 'If that's what he wants to do, then fair play to him,' my Dad said.

The majority of the management and team were there when I arrived at Na Fianna, all in good spirits naturally. I got among my teammates and enjoyed a couple of drinks too. The couple of hours seemed to fly by, and before I knew it, my sister texted me to say she was on her way. I hadn't told anyone I was only planning to stay for a couple of hours, and now I made my way out to my sister in the car park without telling anyone I was going. I knew my absence wouldn't be noticed for a while at least, because of the sheer number of people there. Ironically, I was actually enjoying myself around the time I left.

When I got back home, I started to think I was missing out. There were contrasting voices going on in my head. I should be celebrating and savouring these moments with my teammates, one voice said. You've done the right thing, said another. I went downstairs, a bit confused as to how I should really feel. Looking back at it now with a clear mind, the reality is that I was crippling myself. I was letting the voices in my head take over and rob me of special moments such as these.

I was being congratulated walking around my local area and further afield in the days after the Leinster final. Though I liked to keep to myself, it was nice to have people both young and old come up to me and say complimentary things. On many occasions over the course of that week I felt low in myself, and having people approach me and say those nice things meant a great deal to me.

We learned who our next opponents would be, in the quarter-final of the All Ireland: Monaghan. Regardless of what team you meet in Ulster, you know you're in for a battle right up to the final whistle. If that thought wasn't enough, the prospect of a place in the All Ireland semi-final back in Croke Park also gave an added impetuous to our training in the lead up to the game.

The three-week lead in to this match didn't seem long at all. Having a daily routine to keep me occupied made time fly. I found myself mostly in a good headspace, and every day that went by without any drastic change in mood was very much welcomed. Before we knew it, the final session before the quarter-final was upon us. At this point in the season, it was all about repetition. Nothing we did in the final session was a surprise to us, from the moment we got into the dressing room to the moment Dessie had the final word.

The following day, one day out from the match, I met up with a few friends in the afternoon to kill some time. This worked on two levels – firstly, it kept me from thinking about the match too much; and secondly, it kept me from ruminating about negative things. However, when I got home that evening, I prepared for all eventualities, from the minute I would meet my teammates for the pre-match meal to getting off the bus coming home after the game. The previous three weeks had been the best I had felt mentally so far that year. So much so that I dared to think I could start looking forward again, that perhaps the worst was behind me. Overriding this however was that negative voice, constantly reminding me of the 'what if?'.

I was a big believer in routine in the lead up to a match, and the morning of this match was no different, including my routine breakfast, free time and packing my gear bag. I prepared for all eventualities through the use of visualisation and role play in my head, not knowing how valuable this technique would later be to me. I visualised the pre-match meal, the journey on the bus, the dressing room, the match itself, the post-match meal and the journey on the bus home. I would picture the ideal scenario, in which I felt most comfortable. I also visualised uncomfortable scenarios, and how I would overcame them.

Everything I had visualised for the pre-match meal, the bus journey to Park Esler and the warm up was as close as it could've been to reality, meaning that I had a calm, clear head from the moment I set foot on the pitch. The match was nip and tuck for large parts. In the end though, we managed to get the scores we needed to pull away. There wasn't any over-exuberance in celebrating the victory – of course, there were smiles all round and pats on the back, but the mentality of the group was to regard this as just another step closer.

The excitement did rise a little in the dressing room when we learned who our next opponents would be. Dessie informed us that on 2 September, we would be back in Croke Park to face Kerry. The long-standing tradition of Kerry football is there for everyone to see. These are the kind of matches you dream about as a kid growing up. As if the incentive of being one match away from an All Ireland final wasn't enough, the opportunity to turn over Kerry in the process certainly was.

Normally on the bus home I would have had my earphones in, but the atmosphere in the group and how I was feeling made me want to embrace the moment and be in amongst it all. I arrived home still on cloud nine.

Three weeks time, 2 September. That's all that was on my mind as I struggled to settle into bed that night.

There was a lot happening at this period in my life. With the recommencement of school, I would have to juggle my Leaving Certificate year with preparing for an All Ireland semi-final. I liked to keep busy though, and keep myself distracted. The more I did the better, for the time being anyway. I wasn't overly studious, but at the same time, I wanted to do well in the Leaving Certificate. I was looking forward to going back to school. I hadn't seen many of my classmates or friends during the summer. The teachers who took an interest in my sporting life congratulated me on my achievements over the summer.

The week of the All Ireland semi-final coincided with the recommencement of school. Training had gone well over the last two weeks. Collectively and personally preparations were going well on the field for the lead up to the game.

I started to struggle off the field again though. I thought returning to school and settling back into a routine I was familiar with would be the ideal thing for me, as a person and sporting wise. I guess I didn't prepare myself enough for the perceptions of others – that I was something of a celebrity, supposedly living this idyllic life. Over the summer, I was used to waking up and not feeling myself on certain days, but I had had time to myself to sort it out before going about my day. Suddenly, I didn't have that freedom anymore. On a couple of mornings in our first week back, I didn't quite feel myself, but I found I didn't have time in the morning to deal with whatever was going on in my head.

Then, students and teachers constantly telling me how they'd love to be in my shoes, preparing for an All Ireland semi-final in Croke Park in just under a week's time, didn't help either. Of course, this wasn't the students' or teachers' fault. They weren't to know the inner turmoil I was going through. They didn't know that some mornings I put up a front, pretending everything was okay when it really wasn't. All they saw was a popular, smiling individual who looked to be living an idyllic life.

The school week came to an end. On my short drive home, I should have been looking forward to the game against Kerry in two days' time, but I wasn't. The weight I had felt on my shoulders in school throughout that day was making its way home with me. I tried to visualise defeating Kerry on the Sunday and playing a pivotal role in the process. I managed to envisage exactly that, but failed to attach any positive emotion to it.

At home, everything seemed dark and dreary. My head felt like it weighed a ton, as I struggled to pick it up from between my legs. I must have spent an hour in this position, going into a spiral of negative emotions. Scooby was due to collect me for training in a matter of hours. My parents and sister still weren't home from work yet. As I got my gear ready, I was exhausted trying to fight the way I felt.

My parents arrived home. Whether I liked it or not, I had to muster up the energy again to put up a front, because the idea of telling them how I was feeling hadn't even crossed my mind. In reality, it was probably a good thing that my parents walked through the door, because I was immersed in a never-ending negative spiral. I chatted to my parents until Scooby arrived.

All I wanted to do was go out onto the pitch and forget about the day I had had. Out there, I struggled to get up to the pitch of excitement my teammates were at, but I soon felt a hell of a lot better than I had for the majority of the day. Scooby and I were named to line out in midfield again for what would be our biggest game to date. We discussed various things about the match in the car on the way home, but truthfully, my mind was elsewhere. I wanted to get home, get into bed and forget about the day I had just had. I hoped the following day would bring better fortune.

As I rose from my bed the next morning, I didn't feel the weight of the world on my shoulders anymore. I just felt strangely numb. The prospect of eating breakfast and getting ready to meet my friends for a couple of hours neither excited me or got me feeling down. It was as if the conveyor belt of emotions was jammed – there just wasn't anything coming out. The thought of the match the following day evoked the same numbness.

Nothing changed throughout the day. Even when I got some alone time that evening, I was stuck in a trance, confused as to how I should feel. It had been a bizarre last twenty-four hours. Anyone would think I had the world at my feet. One day out from the biggest match I would play in my career to date, yet I felt nothing. The unpredictability of my own emotions scared me.

The following morning, match day, as I leaned over to switch off my alarm, my first thought was, 'This is the day.' I felt butterflies in my stomach, and I was immensely glad that I could feel once more. I felt nervous about letting myself get excited about the match, but I did, I went there and it felt amazing. I went about my usual match-day morning routine, and had a chat with my dad. I tried to avoid any conversation about football, but that's always hard in the presence of my dad, such is his love for the game.

Scooby arrived, and I hugged my parents as they wished us good luck. Scooby was in good spirits on the way to DCU. The routine was the same as usual, including seating arrangements on the bus as we departed DCU for Croke Park. I listened to the same playlist as I had before the previous matches, right down to listening to the same song at the same landmark as all the times before.

At the ground, everything was the same as for the Leinster final. The prize was that bit bigger this time though, and I couldn't wait to be amongst it all. After a walk of the pitch, taking it all in for a few minutes, I headed back down the steps of the Cusack Stand and into the dressing room. Everyone's usual pre-match rituals were going on before the collective warm up. I was a man of few superstitions, but I would always put on my right sock before my left, and my right glove before my left. The indoor warm up complete. Dessie said his final words before we emerged from the tunnel.

The crowd was noticeably larger than for the Leinster final. However, once you get going on the pitch, all of that goes from the forefront of your mind. After the week I had had, and particularly the last few days, I was glad to be out in the place where I always felt most happy. The national anthem was belted out, and we took our positions on the field of play. Then the match was underway, and there was no place I'd rather have been. For the next sixty minutes I was fully focused.

As expected, the game came right down to the wire. The confidence we had built up all year to finish out games strongly stood to us yet again. Coming down the closing stages, we tagged on the vital scores that would eventually see us out as victors. As the final whistle was blown, sheer delight flooded across my teammates and I. We had achieved the goal we had set out early on in the year – to be there on All Ireland final day.

To really put the icing on the cake, I was taken aside to be awarded Man of the Match. I did manage to enjoy that moment and the celebrations that ensued in the dressing room. However, when the conversation began about where we would celebrate that night, the voice coming from my shoulder yet again quashed any thought of me joining up with the rest of my teammates. The fear of my emotional state changing at the flick of a switch was too much for me to ignore. Even though I was in a good headspace at that moment, having just won a place in the All Ireland final, and being awarded Man of the Match too, I didn't know whether I could go out and enjoy my night. The familiar doubts, the 'what if?' feelings, played on my mind. 'What if my mood changes and I break down in front of everyone?' I worried.

Regardless of how good I was feeling, the fear of that was too much. I told Scooby as he dropped me home that I wouldn't make it out, as I was just worn out from the whole day. I gave the same excuse to my family as we sat down to relax for the evening, in the safety of home.

The All Ireland final was now three weeks away. We were due to face Meath, for the third time that year. My life during this time consisted of going to school and training. If I had an evening off from training, I went up to the club to practise my free kicks. Club members of all ages would come up to me in the middle of my sessions to wish me good luck. A banner was even hung outside the local leisure centre wishing me good luck. I was genuinely touched by all the well-wishers and the gestures of support, and I felt a responsibility to deliver my best performance yet come All Ireland final day. There was pressure, especially as interest levels among the general public had taken a spike, but as always, I found training a massive release.

My mood fluctuated, as it had since January. When people approached me, with the best of intentions, to tell me how lucky I was and how great it must be to be involved in such an occasion, I struggled to deal with it at times. I worried that I should have felt the way they did for me, but I simply couldn't. I could take my mind to the build up surrounding the All Ireland final, to the match itself and, if it was to be, to the celebrations that would follow. But I couldn't attach any positive emotion to it. I was bemused at this, and found myself in a negative spiral, blaming myself for feeling this way. I relied on training to give me the release I needed.

In the week of the game, I was never too far away from a conversation about it. Dessie and all the backroom team had done an incredible job of making us feel like it was only another game. 'We play the game, not the occasion,' I recall Dessie saying. We were constantly reminded that what we had done previously to get us this far had worked – nothing away from that needed to be attempted.

The only place I wanted to be was on the training field. You can imagine then that I was only too delighted to exit the school gates on Friday afternoon. At this stage mentally I was feeling okay. I didn't get overly excited about the impending final, but I was glad I was in a relatively good headspace for the time being. Our last session that evening was like any other, two days out from a game. The same team that had started the semi-final against Kerry was named again for the final. It was a proud moment for myself, my family, my club and my friends. I wanted to keep everything the same in the lead up to this game too. Routine had served me well up to this point, so the next day, I followed the same routine as I had for the semi-final and the games before that. It was hard to keep the thought of the game out of my head, but I was happy that the dark clouds were well out of sight. I went to bed relaxed and woke up in the same manner.

Everyone in your circle has a part to play in the build up to a big game, and there was no bigger game than this one. Any doubt as to whether my emotional state would hold up took a back seat for the time being. I was immersed in visualising how I would ideally like the game to pan out, both personally and collectively. Between getting my gear ready and my breakfast, this is what I occupied my mind with, and it seemed to make the time go that bit faster.

The drive with Scooby, the pre-match meal, the bus journey, the dressing room, the walk on the pitch, the indoor warm up – we went through it all mechanically, like déjà vu. I can't speak for my other teammates, because everyone's experience is different on All Ireland final day, but I had very much bought into the concept of 'just another game'.

You would sometimes hear from players and fans that there was something magic in the air. Well, if there was, I blocked that out as well. Only upon reflection do you get the full view of what it was like during the on-field warm up, the national anthem and the game itself. At the time, it all seems to blend into one. You get so drawn in by the whole occasion that it almost feels like an out-of-body experience.

We had the upper hand for much of the game, though that wasn't fully reflected on the scoreboard. We were leading by five points at half time, but that lead was narrowed very soon after the half time interval, when Meath cut the margin down to one point. However, we finally regained a stranglehold on the game, and came out as six-point victors.

My abiding memory when the whistle went was embracing both Ross McGowan and Scooby in the middle of the pitch. A great wave of emotions washed over us all in the moments thereafter. David Byrne, our captain, was presented with the Tom Markham trophy, and we all took turns lifting the coveted trophy in triumph. Celebrations continued in the dressing room, and long into the night. We had achieved what we had set out to do, and I was thrilled to have played a pivotal role in our victory. I managed to keep my demons at bay for the vast majority of the traditional week-long celebrations that followed all over Dublin. At moments during this week, I thought I saw a little hint of light at the end of the tunnel, which I hoped would shine brighter in the following days and weeks.

When the dust had finally settled on the final and all the celebrations slowed down, it was time to return to normal life. Since the beginning of January, as a Dublin footballer, your mind is focused solely on winning the All Ireland. Nothing else matters. Of course other things go on besides football, but you are in a bubble the majority of the time – a bubble that only the thirty-plus panel members and management team are in.

Now, in the off season, I desperately wanted to create my own bubble. Any form of physical activity was me entering that bubble. When I was doing physical exercise, I could be myself, I didn't have to put up a front. The release of happy endorphins made me feel like I was worth something, when my mind wanted me to feel otherwise.

I settled into my new routine and, for the most part, was getting by each day without any major problems going on in my head. On a typically wet and cold October's day, a month after the All Ireland final, I had just got a haircut in the local village when I received a phone call. On the other end of the line was Michael 'Deego' Deegan. I knew Deego already as his son, named Michael too, was on my team in the season gone by. He quite quickly let me know what he was ringing about. Jim Gavin had recently been appointed Dublin senior football manager, and Deego told me that he was going to be part of his management team for the upcoming 2013 campaign. Jim wanted me up for the beginning of the 2013 campaign, with a view to being part of the panel should I do well in the early stages.

I paused for a moment, eyes and mouth wide open, trying to register what had just been said to me. I composed myself enough to respond with, 'Okay, that's great.' This was a fairly low-key response to such earth-shattering news, an opportunity I could only dream of. As I gathered myself some more, Deego said I should expect a text message over the coming days to inform me where and when the first meeting would be held. The phone call ended, and I stared at the ground in utter disbelief for a moment.

The first person I rang was my dad. He couldn't quite believe it either. Not that he ever doubted my ability, but it caught us both by surprise that it had happened so early on in my career. Over the next few days, I was congratulated by text or in person by many people that my dad had clearly told.

News travelled fast, and before I knew it, everyone in the local area with even a vague interest in Gaelic football was aware of the news. At eighteen years of age, I had just won my first All Ireland medal, and had been called up to the Dublin senior football team. The spotlight shone ever more brightly over me. This made the next month, leading up to my first meeting with the senior footballers, even more difficult for me from a mental health standpoint.

This first meeting was at the end of November in Parnell Park. I was in school earlier that day. Naturally, with it being my Leaving Certificate year, there was a lot going on. All I could think about though was the meeting that evening, with players I had watched from the stands and idolised for many years. The hairs on the back of my neck stood up at the thought of it, and a smile stretched across my face.

I could share my excitement in the car on the way to the meeting with my clubmate Kevin O'Brien, who was also part of the panel. Kevin had been involved in the senior panel since the year before, so I threw question after question at him. As we parked up and made our way upstairs to the meeting room, I went very quiet. My heart was beating out of my chest, and I was fidgeting at my trouser pockets and the strings from my jumper.

We entered the room, where lads were standing around and chatting. Among them were the likes of Paul Flynn, Bernard Brogan and Stephen Cluxton. I knew some in the group from playing with or against them at club level. Soon, Jim Gavin came into the room and the meeting commenced. I sat in the middle row at the very right-hand side of the room. Every so often, I'd look to the left of me and spot even more players that I had watched on television. I checked in with myself on numerous occasions during the course of the meeting, thinking, 'Is this really happening?' The meeting soon came to a close, and Jim quickly went around and shook every player's hand to welcome them. I was still in a state of shock getting back into the car.

That evening, I filled my family in on how the meeting went and what it was like to be in the room with so many idols of mine. My friends, of course, kept asking me all about it in school in the days following the meeting. The first training session was only a couple of weeks away, and I simply couldn't wait.

Everything then from the outside looking in seemed like it was going right for me in my life. I had a loving family, who were behind me in everything I did; I was popular among friends; I had recently won my first All Ireland medal; and, at the tender age of eighteen, I had been drafted into the Dublin senior set up. However, everything was not as it seemed. I was still going through a battle in my head on a daily basis. It seemed like the more I was achieving, the less likely I was to come out and tell people what I was going through. The mask that I had been wearing for some time now was becoming almost second nature. In moments that I had to myself around this time, when I could take down the mask and be vulnerable, I kept asking myself, 'Why, why, why?' The idyllic life that everyone could see I was living? I could see it too. The problem was that I couldn't make contact with the positive emotions that should have stemmed from it.

My first training session with the senior team was a prime example of this. I thought that if I didn't show the same level of excitement as I had for the meeting in Parnell Park, Kevin might question whether something was up with me. I had to put up a front on the way to training with him. I wish I could have talked about how surreal it was to train with the Dublin senior footballers for the first time – how it felt to share a dressing room with these players I idolised, the time I touched shoulders with Kevin McManamon before the beginning of the bleep test, or having a post-session meal sitting with Kevin Nolan and Michael Darragh MacAuley. All of these things happened, but my mind simply couldn't let me enjoy those moments, because it was stuck elsewhere, in troubled waters.

I was not only lying to myself, but I was lying to others around me. I was telling my family and friends what an unforgettable moment it was to train with the senior team for the first time, something that would 'last with me forever'. Part of this was true – I wouldn't forget it – but I made out that it was one of the happiest and proudest moments of my life to date. In the following weeks, as training proceeded with the senior team, I continued to extend that lie to anyone who asked me how training was going.

Even though I was having difficulties in my everyday life, my performances on the pitch never dipped. Yes, I was still in a negative headspace right up to the moment when I was sitting in the dressing room before training, but once I stepped over that white line, all my troubles were left behind. My performances on the pitch led to my inclusion for the National League campaign, which began in January, a year into my journey with depression. My first appearance in the National League didn't go without a mishap however.

In the week leading up to the first National League game, I had a Dublin 'A' schools final on the Wednesday. Unfortunately, things didn't go our way and we lost the match. The following evening, we were due to have our final session before the first League game, against Cork in Croke Park that Saturday night. I was given the night off training, having played the previous day. I watched on from the sidelines, and joined the squad upstairs afterwards for a meeting and the team announcement.

As Jim announced the team, I noticed that my name wasn't on the board. I hadn't made the squad. I was disappointed, but had to recognise the strength in depth he had at his disposal. I went home that evening to tell my parents I wouldn't be involved in the first League game. My dad told me, 'This is all a learning curve. You're very young, and you just have to bide your time with all of it.'

Saturday arrived and I hadn't made many plans. I headed into Malahide, where I decided to get my hair cut. Then I went down the road to get a Starbucks. While I was in getting my coffee, my phone rang. It was Shane O'Hanlon, Jim's right-hand man. He asked where I was, and I told him. He told me they had made a mistake, and had meant to include me in the substitutes list. In a blind panic, I rushed back home to get my gear. I didn't have time to register that this was going to be my first involvement for the seniors in the League, as it all happened too quickly.

Luckily, my dad was at home to give me a lift. As I was running late and the team would be leaving the Gibson hotel shortly to drive to Croke

Park, Shane had told me the bus would meet me along the way, on East Wall Road. My dad dropped me off a few minutes ahead of the bus. I waited there nervously, tracksuit on and gear bag in hand. My heart rate had increased, and I couldn't stand easy. I was preparing myself for the inevitable slagging that would come my way when I stepped onto the bus.

The bus pulled up and I got on. Apart from the odd jeer or two as I took my seat near the front of the bus, everyone seemed fine, completely focused on the game ahead. I had over-thought the whole situation. This was an example of how out of touch I was with my emotional balance around this time. I didn't have the skills and coping mechanisms to assess a situation rationally.

The night ended on a positive note. I made my first National League appearance, coming off the bench for the final ten minutes of the game.

I had a lot on my plate, with training the school year in full swing. I would go to the gym for 6.30am on a Tuesday and Thursday. I'd go from there to school, where oftentimes I'd be a bit late for the first class of the morning. I'd arrive home from school just after 4pm every day, and attempt to get any bit of homework or study done that I could in the time that I had. I'd be out the door again at about 6pm to go to training. It was a lot to contend with, but I never once wished that the pace of my life would slow down, because I loved to be busy. And the main reason I loved to be busy was to keep my mind distracted.

Things weren't getting any better for me from a mental health point of view. When I would walk into the first class late, people in the class would remark, 'Don't worry, everyone, Shane's late because he was just at Dublin training.' I would plant a big smile on my face as I made my way to my seat, but this was in stark contrast to how I was really feeling. I had a lot of thinking time by myself in the car from Blanchardstown, where we trained, back to school in Portmarnock. On many occasions, I took the longest possible route back to school, while I tried to get my head to a level where I could function in front of my classmates. I often went into spirals of negative thought, some deeper than others.

For anyone who hasn't experienced a negative thought spiral, it can be hard to understand. Firstly, a negative thought comes into your head. You then focus on that negative thought, filtering your experiences through this negative filter. Positive events are therefore made negative too. Negative thinking causes a negative feeling, which causes more negative experiences, which causes more negative thoughts, hence a negative spiral. This often went on for the whole car journey. When I eventually did arrive at the school car park, I'd sometimes need another few minutes in the car to compose myself before putting up that mask and facing everyone. There was no end to how low I could feel, it seemed. Still though, my crutch was sport, and I would rely on it more than ever in the coming months.

It was now coming up to April. Football was going relatively well up to then. I had made a few more appearances in the League and gained vital experience over this time. We reached the League final, when we would face Tyrone. This would be a busy few weeks – not only did I have the League final to contend with, but I also had the small matter of sitting my Leaving Certificate German and Irish oral exams around this time. Sitting down to prepare for my orals wasn't an issue. Much like my fifth year exams the previous year, I found studying a welcome distraction. The difference between my two main coping mechanisms, however, was that I didn't get the same release of endorphins from studying as I did from exercise. In order to sit down and study, I had to be in a stable frame of mind, whereas I often went out to exercise while I was in the depths of despair, and it helped me to get out of the rut I was in.

One day I got into difficulty trying to study in an unstable mind frame. It was the day before my German oral exam. Moe and I were in the same German class. We wanted to get away from studying for a couple of hours, so we organised to meet up in the evening, with Karl too, in Pavillions shopping centre. All that day, I had felt out of sorts. From the moment I left my bed, I didn't feel myself. I hadn't been feeling myself for well over a year now, but this was something I hadn't quite experienced yet.

I had sat in school all that day, exhausted. Keeping up a front constantly was taking a real toll on me now. I recall going to the toilet between almost every class. I locked myself away in the cubicle for a few minutes each time, sat down on the toilet and buried my head in my hands. My hands covered my eyes, which made everything dark on the outside, reflecting how I felt inside. All through the day I was on the cusp of drowning, admitting defeat. I trudged along the school corridors, feeling like each step was heavier than the one before. For the first time, I felt like this dull, bleak, hopeless feeling wasn't going to leave me.

The school day finally came to an end, and all I wanted to do was crawl into bed and shut off from absolutely everything. The smallest of tasks exhausted me – turning the key to the front door, walking up the stairs, taking off my uniform – they all seemed to take a huge effort. I lay in bed feeling like I had the weight of the world on top of me. I fell asleep shortly after my head hit the pillow.

I woke up almost three hours later, having completely forgotten about my plans with Karl and Moe. I looked at my phone – unsurprisingly, there were three missed calls from Karl, obviously wondering where I was. It was coming up to 7pm, an hour after we were to meet. I gave the excuse that I had left my phone downstairs while studying for my oral exam, and hadn't noticed the time going by. I said I was going to stay in for the night and get more study in.

The dull, bleak, hopeless feeling that had enveloped me for most of the day had subsided somewhat. However, I still felt mentally drained. This made sitting down to actually do some preparation for the following day's exam extremely difficult.

The following day, I was very nervous as I sat outside the exam room, waiting to be called. I hadn't prepared in the way that I wanted, which added to the anxiety that naturally comes with a State exam anyway. I went in and surprised myself with how well it went. I let out a big sigh of relief coming out of the exam room. I had gotten away with it on this particular day, but the way I was living my life wasn't healthy and it most certainly wasn't normal.

Two weeks passed, and it was time to sit my Irish oral exam. In comparison with the German oral, my preparation was much easier. Everything in my body felt light, my mind felt active and I was energetic and enthusiastic, hoping to do well in the exam.

For well over a year now, I had been experiencing these peaks and troughs in my mood. I was ignorant of the fact that I needed help. Every time my mood lifted and I was feeling good, I would tell myself that I had turned a corner and the worst was behind me. My subconscious knew I was masking the truth though. Yes, I did slip in and out of low moods, but they were getting progressively worse and more debilitating. I clearly didn't want to face up to the elephant in the room, so I just got on with things. I sat my Irish oral, and I was fairly happy with how it went.

The League final came at the end of April, in what was a hectic few weeks. I was named on the bench and hoped to have a part to play. Preparations were much like for the minors. We met a few hours before the game in the Gibson hotel, off Dublin's north quays. This is where we would always meet for games in Croke Park. Just like with the minors, we would have our pre-match meal and pre-match brief before getting on the bus for the stadium. Specific seating arrangements were also a thing with the seniors.

At Croke Park, our dressing room was at the Hogan Stand side of the ground, where for the minors it was on the Cusack Stand side. The media presence was slightly larger now, as were the dressing rooms and warm up area. These were all subtle differences, nothing too big to deter us from focusing on the game.

This being the League final also didn't change anything in our preparation. Everything was like clockwork – Jim's mantra was repetition, repetition, repetition. We arrived in the dressing room, checked what number jersey we had for the day, took our seats underneath our jerseys, then took twenty minutes to ourselves, to do our own thing – some went out to watch the game that was on before ours, some did a preliminary warm up, some listened to music and others stood around chatting. Then came the indoor warm up, lasting about ten minutes, and then we went back into the dressing room to get any last bits we needed before Jim's final briefing. Finally, we went out onto the pitch to do the final bit of warm up before game time.

Starting on the bench, as I did for the entirety of the League, I tried to focus on players in my position, what they were doing well and what I could potentially exploit should I come on. It was good that I did do that, because at half time with the game level at ten points each, I was called upon. I remember my clubmate Kevin O'Brien patting me on the back and saying, 'Let's see you now,' as we made our way out onto the pitch for the second half. He probably meant it as the most innocuous gesture, but for me it wasn't. I was going through a multitude of thoughts, from the past to the future and back, but that small pat on the back and word from Kevin made me slip right into the present moment.

Thankfully, once the ball was thrown up for the start of the second half, any other thoughts disappeared and I was fully immersed in the contest. It was a tight game right the way through, but in the end we came out victors by the smallest of margins, 0-18 to 0-17. Deego, our selector, made a beeline for me, embracing me in sheer delight. After that, the whole aftermath was a bit of a blur. At such a young age, to have been called upon and trusted in to make an impact – it was a very proud moment. It was a nice feeling to walk up the steps of the Hogan Stand in front of 33,000 supporters, to lift my first trophy at senior level.

The pedestal that people saw me as standing on grew even larger as a result of our win. I was able to handle the expectation that people had of me, especially in school and around my area, when my mind was right. The day after the League final, the moment I set foot in the school, I had class-mates and students from all year groups coming up to congratulate me. I was humbled. Mr O'Ceara, the school GAA manager, shouted my name – 'Shane, Shane, Shane!' – and made his way across a hall full of students to me. I ended up being late for class because he kept me talking for twenty minutes, which I didn't mind at all.

Numerous times over the coming weeks, people stopped me in school or on the street to have a chat. The usual theme was, 'You're so lucky to have everything you have going for you, and at such a young age too!' I was fine with people saying that about me. To be honest, it was true – I was very lucky to be in my position, and all of it so early in my life. I was truly blessed.

Issues only began to arise when I experienced my low episodes. I felt I couldn't be seen to express how I truly felt on the inside. This depressed, hopeless character, who couldn't find any joy in what he was doing, simply couldn't be seen on the outside. That made the upcoming summer my most difficult yet. I had to get my Leaving Certificate out of the way before I could solely focus on what I hoped would be a long summer of football. In the meantime, I wanted to be involved in football all the way up to the start of the exams. My last involvement in football before a short break was against Westmeath in the first round of the Leinster Championship. We came out on top, winning 1-22 to 0-09. Ten days later, I sat my first exam.

Anyone who has sat the Leaving Certificate will know all about the crash you experience after each exam. Hand cramps, creaks in your neck, cramps mid-exam and overall stiffness in your body from being in a fixed position for hours at a time are all part of it too. You can imagine then my joy after finishing the third day of exams and having the weekend off to recharge.

That joy was short-lived, however, because not long after arriving home from my exam, I felt my mood change for the worse. That low, dark, dreary feeling came for a visit again. I didn't let it sit with me for too long though. I wanted to be proactive and fight against it. I went straight to my usual crutch – exercise. No sooner did those negative feelings come over me than I was out the door in my running gear, hood up and headphones on. What better place was there to go on a warm, sunny summer's evening than the beach? For the next few hours, it was just me, my music and the picturesque curve of Portmarnock beach.

I relied on exercise to keep me afloat through the remainder of my exams, because nothing else I tried seemed to work. I met up with friends over the weekend, but this just left me feeling more mentally fatigued. My mind wouldn't let me tap into the positive feelings I would usually get from time with friends. Yet again, I had to put up a front on the outside, while the demons were slowing chipping away, getting deeper and deeper inside.

I tried visualisation, which had also worked for me in the past. I focused on the thing that gave me the most joy – football, of course. I imagined walking into the dressing room for the first time after finishing my exams; being out on the training pitch; laughing and joking with teammates; and running out into Croke Park on Championship Sunday. I could visualise all of this vividly. I saw myself standing tall and proud; walking back into the dressing room, beaming from ear to ear; training with my teammates; and loving every moment of running out into a packed Croke Park.

Seeing it wasn't the problem. It was feeling the associated emotions that I couldn't manage. I sat at the edge of my bed, head downwards staring at the wooden floor, slouched over with my hands on my knees, wishing that the Shane I was visualising could feel that way right now.

One thing that helped was running. I went out running every day during the remainder of my exams. I organised my study times around it. I figured I'd be most enthusiastic about studying after a run, so that's what I did. My parents didn't question my daily run – they were unaware that the major reason for it was to escape my inner turmoil, which showed no sign of going away any time soon.

By the end of my exams, I was absolutely exhausted, as most people are. Not only had I to contend with the huge mental fatigue that the Leaving Certificate naturally brings, but I had to put up a mask to make it look like everything was great in my life, day after day, and this took a huge toll on me too. The fear of people finding out what was going on in my mind trumped any thought I had of letting my guard down and allowing myself to be vulnerable.

My exams eventually came to a close, which brought some measure of relief. While everyone else went out on the last night of the exams, I was off training with the Dublin team. It was hardly a thing to be complaining about – any young, aspiring footballer would have jumped at the prospect of training with the Dublin senior team. I was very aware of the lucky position I was in, but my inability to attach joy to anything left me feeling numb.

A week after finishing the exams, I was out with Moe for a coffee. We chatted about the summer ahead, and he mentioned a few music festivals that he was thinking of going to. He was also going to enjoy going out for drinks during the week or at the weekend, without the worry of exams hanging over him, and of course there was the infamous sixth year holiday coming up at the start of August, taking place in Magaluf this year. When he threw the question back to me, my answer was, 'A long summer of football, with hopefully a bit of silverware at the end of it.'

Moe asked, 'Do you ever think how many other eighteen-year-olds would love to be in the position you're in right now?' 'Yeah,' I said, breaking into a fake smile while getting an empty feeling in the pit of my stomach. That same question stuck with me everywhere I went throughout the summer, as I struggled to regain any hope of feeling normal again.

Football continued, and I fought a losing battle as the days and weeks wore on. At the end of June, we defeated Kildare in the Leinster semi-final, setting up a date with Meath two weeks later, when we would battle it out to be crowned Leinster Champions. Admittedly, coming back into the team after a few weeks off, I was a bit off the pace, which meant I didn't travel with the team for the semi-final. That gave me a focus to get back fitter and sharper, to put my hand up for selection for the next occasion.

I was in search of a job for the summer – to gather up a bit of money, but also to give me a structure and routine so that I wouldn't be sitting at home ruminating all day. I remembered how having a routine the previous summer had helped me a great deal. At the start of July, I started to hand out CVs to various shops and businesses in the area.

I mentioned this to Kevin on the way to training one of the evenings, and he told me to get in touch with Stephen 'Shocko' O'Shaughnessy, who was in charge of the Dublin development camps. Shocko was holding the Dublin GAA development camp in mid-July for the fourteen to sixteen year olds in the Dublin development squads. I hadn't realised that all the coaches were from the Dublin senior panel, including Kevin. I rang Shocko that evening after training, and he was more than happy to have me on board. The camp was due to begin the day after the Leinster final.

The team for the Leinster final was announced, as always, on the Friday before the game. My reward for performing relatively well in training for the last number of weeks was inclusion in the squad. All was not well however. On the Saturday, the day before the game, I had arranged to meet up with friends. I would spend most of my morning and early afternoon lounging around the house, watching whatever sport was on the television, then meet up with Karl and go to the driving range, followed by some food.

My plans changed as soon I woke on Saturday morning. The dark cloud descended and the inner dialogue started up again. What reason had I to be feeling like this? A relaxing morning lay ahead, followed by time with my friend, and not to forget a Leinster final to look forward to in just over twenty-four hours. None of this excited me in the least. My rational mind told me this was all great, but very quickly my irrational mind stormed in and quashed any positive associations with this thought. Inside my mind, I was screaming at this irrational voice, 'Stop, stop, go away!' I couldn't control it though; I hadn't the tools to combat it.

I tried to go about my morning, in the hope that this inner voice would quieten down. In the kitchen, my dad and sister were making breakfast. A conversation was going on between them, but I couldn't tune in – it felt like any time I tried to engage in what was going on around me, my mind would pull me back into a great pool of negative emotion. I didn't stay in the kitchen long, as I was anxious that they would notice me going into a trance every few moments. I had to get out of the house.

I went upstairs to get changed. Everything felt panicked. My eyes couldn't settle on one thing, my head turning to a different position every couple of seconds. I was opening drawers, pulling out clothes from my wardrobe in a blind panic. When I eventually managed to get dressed, I couldn't stop ruffling at my clothes. I quickly dashed out of the house and got into the car. I didn't know where I was going, but I found myself heading towards Portmarnock train station car park. This is a pretty big car park, and I drove down toward the back, where there were no other cars. I turned off the engine, music still playing in the background, still fidgeting with my clothes and everything around me. Tears began to well up inside me.

For a year and a half now, I've been holding the tears back. How have I gotten to this point? I asked myself. Why can't I get away from this crippling feeling? These questions brought no answers, just more confusion. Soon, I broke into tears and did nothing to hold them back. I felt utterly useless, defeated. I anxiously looked around, hoping no one was coming near as the tears fell from me. I was past breaking point. Eighteen years of age and everything going for me, and here I was, a defeated and broken man.

I wept for hours in that car park, as a deep sense of hopelessness took hold of my body. I was a shell of a man when I eventually brought my head up to peer into the rear-view mirror – I was pale and exhausted-looking, with bloodshot eyes. The tears dried up but I sat for another long while, until my eyes and face looked normal again. I sent a message to Karl saying I wouldn't be around, as I'd forgotten I'd already made plans with my sister, Stephanie. Of course, this was untrue. I went home and sat in for the evening, exhausted from the afternoon's reckonings.

The mask was put on the following day, Leinster final day. My team-mates were none the wiser as I arrived at the Gibson hotel in what looked like good spirits, looking forward to the contest ahead. We managed to get over the line by seven points, and this limelight figure with everything going right in his life was yet again up on the Hogan Stand steps, this time to lift the Delaney cup. The celebrations started back in the Gibson hotel, and continued out into the city centre.

The development camps came at the right time. I knew the coming weeks were going to be challenging, having entered a new stage in my continuing depressive episodes. However, if there was anything I'd learnt from the previous eighteen months, it was that I needed to keep busy to stay out of the never-ending cycle of dark moods. After the highs and lows of the weekend just past, all I wanted to do was engage in my new coaching role, along with preparing for the All Ireland quarter-final at the beginning of August.

I felt a degree of pressure walking into the dressing rooms at DCU for the start of the development camps. Eight Dublin senior footballers, including myself, were introduced by Shocko to the fifty young, aspiring footballers that we would have the pleasure of coaching over the coming weeks. Every one of them gazed up at us, hanging on to every last word we said as we each made a short introduction. The poker face I was so used to putting on would have to be absolutely bulletproof around this group of players – they would be watching our every move, from how we carried ourselves, how we walked, how we talked and how we coached. Any chink in my exterior would open me to questions that I didn't want to answer. The most challenging part of it was when players were given a chance to ask questions. Not surprisingly, they asked what it was like to be on the Dublin senior team, what our training was like, who our best player was, what it was like to run out in front of 82,500 fans, all of that sort of thing. I had to lie to them, to tell them how great it all was. If I had told them that winning the All Ireland with the minors and the National League and Leinster Championship with the seniors coincided with the darkest days of my life, they'd never have believed me. The fear of being judged for feeling this way wasn't worth it. The constant lie that I was living was being reinforced further.

The All Ireland quarter-final was just around the corner now, and our opposition would be Cork. The 'business end' of the Championship was about to begin. No slip ups, no second chances, we had one opportunity to reach the All Ireland semi-final. The intensity at training was something I had never experienced before – thirty players fighting tooth and nail to be included in the twenty-six-man squad that would represent Dublin on 3 August.

The week before the match, we played an internal game, as we did all summer in the lead up to a Championship match. These matches were always fiery. Sometimes tempers flared and it spilled over, but that was all part of being a Dublin footballer. This type of game, this high-octane, pressured environment, gave me the release that I so desperately needed from the ongoing battle in my head.

I had a conversation with Paul Flynn during our post-match meal that day. Paul, a senior figure in the dressing room, was conveying a message to me about what it meant to play for Dublin and the privileged position we all found ourselves in. When he said, 'These are the best days of our lives,' I almost felt guilty. Although I knew exactly what he meant, I was experiencing quite the opposite. I wanted to feel this way, but my mind wouldn't let me.

In the days after that conversation, Paul's 'best days of our lives' comment rang loud in my head. I was now at the point where I had started to hate myself. Before this point, I had wanted to place blame on anything and everything around me for the way I was feeling, but now, eighteen months in, I concluded that I had no one to blame but myself for feeling this way.

I found the build up to the Cork match my most difficult yet. The business end of the season brings more attention to you as a player. No matter where you go, you're never far away from a conversation about the upcoming game. I was used to this on a smaller scale, from the previous two years with the minors. However, senior football is a massive step up in every sense. The previous year, I had had to try to live up to the role of a charmed youngster, living an idyllic life. Now, a year later, even more people saw me as even more blessed, yet the level of depression I was experiencing was on a much deeper level. As time went on, the perception people had of me and the actual reality of my situation seemed to be growing further and further apart.

It was now six days until the All Ireland quarter-final. I had gotten home from coaching at the development camp. I was worn out and just wanted to switch off before preparing for the evening's gym session. The dull, dark, dreary feeling I'd experienced the day before the Leinster final came upon me again as I sat down on the couch in the sitting room. My ability to fight off these depressive episodes was at an all-time low now. The panic that I experienced when I last felt like this wasn't there this time. I slumped over in my chair, head bowed down to the floor and hands on my knees, as I took a deep inhalation followed by an even longer exhalation.

'Here we go again,' I thought. No one was home as the first teardrop hit the floor. The tap was turned on fully as the tears began to flow, gathering beneath me. There was no specific reason why I broke down into a flood of tears. My mind kept taking me through past memories, to times when I was happy. That person felt like he didn't exist anymore. Even when I thought about more recent times, when my mood was lifted and I felt okay, there was always that anxious feeling that my next dip in mood was just around the corner.

The physical release that would help me on this particular evening was in the form of our gym session. I took my frustrations at the way I was feeling out in the session, and felt better for it afterwards. However, on the drive home, I wondered to myself, 'How much longer can I rely on this to keep me afloat?'

I found myself in similar situations twice more that week in the lead up to the game. It felt like I was at the lowest point in my life by the end of the week. The situation looked the complete opposite, as the twenty-six-man squad was announced that Friday with my name at number eighteen. With the week I had just had, you'd think maybe one or two cracks would have begun to show, but this was not the case. My poker face was as bullet proof as ever as I sat into Kevin's car to go to the Gibson hotel that Sunday.

This act continued through the pre-match meal, the warm up and afterwards, when we celebrated getting through to the All Ireland semi-final, having defeated Cork 1-16 to 0-14.

There was a period following our victory against Cork when things didn't feel as dark and dreary as before, though I never got too carried away when I felt somewhat 'normal' again. There were moments around then when my mood did dip and I did feel low, but I felt that it was manageable. It never sank to the depths it had in previous times.

Now, at the beginning of August, my Leaving Certificate results were imminent. I wanted to go to Dublin City University (DCU), to study Sport Science & Health. A man who helped me hugely was Michael Kennedy, who was part of Jim's management team at the time and also Head of Gaelic Games at DCU. When my results came in, he advised me to seek the guidance of Professor Niall Moyna, another man who has played an important role in where I am today. Niall oversaw the Health and Human Performance side of the college, and he advised me on the best path to take. I would first go to Coláiste Dhúlaigh to study General Science for a year, and then begin my Sport Science degree, having built up a bank of knowledge across all science subjects.

This meeting took place in the middle of August, at a time when my mental state was manageable. At a different time, I wouldn't have been able to see the wood for the trees. Niall set out a path that allowed me to see a glimmer of light, a spark of hope that for large periods of the previous eighteen months was missing.

This was all short-lived though. The light I had seen and the hope I had felt were suddenly no longer there. It all changed for me in a matter of days. Even the prospect of an All Ireland semi-final didn't excite me. I began to go back into my shell, fearing that I might never re-emerge again.

I was at such a low point again now that all I could focus my mind on was my very next training session or match. Physical exercise was all I was basing my happiness on. All of the stress, depression and anxiety that were filling my body uncontrollably were at least lessened after a bout of exercise.

I became withdrawn from everybody. When friends asked me to come out somewhere, I made up an excuse each time – usually that I was tired from training and needed to recover at home. I knew from past experience that sitting at home wasn't going to do me any good though. I had two options – either sit at home and be in my head for most of the day, or go out to face the world with a front up. The latter was taking a serious toll on me mentally, so I often chose to stay home, silently wrestling with the inner demons I had little or no control over.

On days when I sat ruminating at home, anxious for the next session to come around, I started to question a lot of things. Was my love for the game really there anymore? I thought back to the same time last year, when my internal struggles were only beginning. I had looked forward to training sessions themselves, but also to the release they gave me afterwards. I was getting to do something I loved, and I was also getting rid of the cloudiness in my head, for a short time at least.

Now, a year later, I gave little thought to the actual training session, but just focussed on the release I'd get from it. Did I care whether it was football, or would any form of exercise do? Once I got that release, it didn't particularly matter. I hated myself for feeling this way. The constant questions that raced around in my head left me with a harshly negative perception of myself.

This continued all the way up to the semi-final. By the time the match came around, I felt like I shouldn't have been there. I was taking away the opportunity from someone else to truly experience the best days of their lives. I had to continue the lie as we overcame Kerry in the semi-final. Another three weeks of pretending that everything in my life was picture-perfect. In reality, I was facing into three weeks of the deepest darkness in my life.

I was introduced to a lot of sports growing up, but Gaelic football was the first sport I fell in love with. I loved everything about it. I remember watching the Dublin team of the 1990s on television with my dad. I remember the first time my dad brought me to watch the 'Dubs' live in Croke Park. I got a taste early on of what it was like to represent Dublin, when I got to put on the famous blue jersey in an under-twelve Easter tournament.

Whether I was playing out in the back garden or in the local GAA club, I would visualise myself running out from beneath the Hogan Stand in front of 82,500 screaming fans on the biggest day of them all – All Ireland final day. Something special is in the air in the week leading up to an All Ireland final. There is a sea of blue everywhere you go. I got a small taste of what this was like as a player with the minor team on All Ireland final day in 2011. The moment Bryan Cullen lifted the Sam Maguire high above his head was etched in my memory, as I thought, 'I'd love to be there one day'.

Now, fast-forward two years; I was seventy minutes away from reaching the pinnacle of my sporting career, and at the tender age of eighteen. People with only the vaguest interest in Gaelic were stopping me on the street to wish me the best. And yet, I was at the lowest point in my life. Why was this? The cloudiness in my head didn't allow me to think rationally and figure it out.

Within the team, there was a lot going on. We had our final internal game, on the top pitch in DCU this time, where we could make use of the floodlights. As Denis Bastick said, 'This is how you know All Ireland final D-day is on the horizon'. This game was the last chance for players to put their hands up to be in contention, especially if you were on the B team, as I was. It was the usual fiery encounter.

Away from the football itself, the ticket frenzy was another issue. Post-match banquet tickets for friends and family were equally as complicated. I was used to such goings-on from the previous two years, but this was on a whole different scale. I went through this time in a daze, in survival mode. Each session was merely getting me through another day.

By the time All Ireland final day came, I was down and out internally. The biggest day of the year on the football calendar, the day that every footballer desperately wants to be a part of – I was one of those lucky ones and yet I was at the lowest point in my life. 'How can this be?' I kept thinking. None of it made sense. I still didn't want anyone to find out what I was going through, but it was hard to keep it together. I felt that the battle-worn mask, that I had done so well to keep up for all this time, was beginning to crack.

I took a deep breath as I opened my bedroom door with my Dublin gear on and gear bag in hand. I made my way down to the kitchen, where my whole family were waiting to wish me well. There were hugs from my mam and my sisters, and a firm handshake and a tight embrace from my dad. 'Do us proud son,' he said as I left. As I closed the front door behind me, the acting performance of my life was about to begin.

I got into Kevin's car and we were on our way to our usual pre-match base, the Gibson hotel. At the hotel, we had our private area where we got to relax and have our pre-match meal. We told ourselves it was 'just another game'. This is what routine, and these familiar surroundings, gave us. Then it was time to get onto the bus, waiting as usual in the underground section of the hotel. Voices in my head were trying to derail my train of thought, which was firmly focused on the match ahead. My headphones were in, playlist chosen and the volume was on full blast in an attempt to drown out any negative thoughts.

The closer we got to the ground, the more supporters we saw. Kids were draped in Dublin's sky-blue, their eyes full of excitement as they caught a glimpse of us driving by. Masses of Dublin and Mayo supporters were shouting and singing as we slowly made our way past. We got into the ground and underneath the stands, out of the public view. We stepped off the bus, keeping our heads down as cameras flashed in our faces until we made it into the dressing room.

As usual, we had some free time before the warm ups, so I went out to catch a bit of the minor final that was in play, before returning to the dressing room to get ready. After our warm up, a final few words of inspiration were delivered by various voices in the dressing room. Jim gave us his final message, and we made our way out from the darkness of the tunnel and into the light.

The roars of 82,500 people echoed all around. The on-field warm up seemed to go by in a flash. I took my seat in the stands and before I knew it the game was underway. As a substitute, it's difficult to watch. It's emotionally and mentally draining. You are constantly watching for potential gaps in the game that you could exploit should you be brought on.

When half time arrived, we went back through the tunnel into the dressing room to regroup. As the players regained their composure, messages were filtered through to each line. Then it was out onto the battlefield again. The second half wore on, and changes were made. I wasn't to be one of them. But that didn't matter one bit when the final whistle was heard and we had come out on top by one point. An almighty roar reverberated around the iconic stadium as players and management flocked onto the field. Grown men were jumping up and down, hugging and kissing one another – this was what it all meant. It was hard to take it all in.

When the chaos on the pitch had settled somewhat, it was time for Stephen Cluxton to lift the Sam Maguire. Another full-blooded roar rose up as he raised the cup above his head. I've often heard sportspeople say that they wish they appreciated moments such as this a bit more than they did as they were happening. This was very much the case for me as I lifted the Sam Maguire cup. Was it all the external stuff away from football that didn't allow me to fully appreciate such a special moment? Or was I simply overawed by the whole occasion?

Celebrations moved from the pitch to the dressing room, and then the Sam Maguire took its place at the front of the bus as we rolled out of Croke Park on our way back to the Gibson hotel for the banquet. I managed to hold it together through the night of celebration with teammates, friends and family. All Ireland final day is an emotional rollercoaster for anyone, never mind having to cover up eighteen months of inner torment.

The celebrations continued throughout the week, and I struggled every step of the way. By the end of the week, I should have been able to look back and smile, knowing that these special moments would live long in the memory, but I couldn't. I wish I could say how special it was to stand on stage with my teammates as thousands of Dublin supporters gathered around Merrion Square to pay tribute. I should be able to say that the hairs were standing up on the back of my neck at that moment. As we emerged onto the stage, I was taken aback by the sheer number of supporters who had turned out – a sea of blue as far as the eye could see. I looked to the left and right of me and every single one of my teammate's mouths was wide open in awe, as they took a few moments to take it all in. I was desperately searching for that feeling too, but it never came. I was left distraught and disillusioned inside, unable to fully engage with what I knew was a momentous occasion.

This continued through the week. At the meet and greet a few days later in Parnell Park, it was the same. We stood in various sections of the pitch, while supporters, young and old, came to get their memorabilia signed. From an external perspective, I had the world at my feet – eighteen years of age and here I was, posing for pictures and signing autographs. Not too long before, I would have been on the other side of that fence, star-struck at meeting players who I idolised.

The fake façade that was in overdrive during all of these celebrations showed no signs of letting up on the Friday of that week. This was a special occasion too – it was my nineteenth birthday. 'What better way to close out an unforgettable week?' everyone said – everyone except me, of course. However, as I had been, I played my part – smiling, bursting with energy and enthusiasm, living my idyllic life. I was telling my friends, who gathered at my house for my birthday, what they wanted to hear. I told them how great it was to lift the Sam Maguire high above my head, to stand out in front of thousands of supporters at Merrion Square, to sign autographs for awestruck fans and to be treated like VIPs all over the city for the entire week.

It was now six days after the All Ireland. The house was quiet, with both my parents and Stephanie gone out for the morning. A dark cloud had been hovering over my head for much of the week gone by, but with the busyness of my schedule I hadn't stopped to think about it. Now, looking back on the week that was meant to be full of ecstasy and happiness, I knew it was anything but. The celebrations that occur over the course of the week after winning an All Ireland will leave you both mentally and physically drained, as the lucky few who have achieved this will tell you. The mental toll it took on me was on a much deeper level though. The battle I had been fighting in my head for almost two years now felt like it was leaning in favour of the dark side, particularly in more recent times. The last week had only served to put another nail in the coffin.

I was now hunched over with my head in my hands, as the tears I had been holding back came streaming out. The negative voice inside of me was taking a firmer grip. Irrational thoughts were spinning around and around in my head. The hope I had held on to now seemed like it was being washed away, that glimmer of light no longer present – the game was over. The negative voice whispered, 'End it all now.'

The first suicidal ideation had now entered my consciousness, and it scared me to the core. My legs shook uncontrollably and I banged my hands on the sides of my head as if to fight away the thought. I stood up in a panic, as if the thoughts in my head might stay where I was sitting. I only made it as far as my bedroom down the hallway before I was hunched over again with my head in my hands. After some time, the tears dried up. Ever so slowly, the inner demons exited my consciousness, but for how long? This was only the start of things to come.

This thing was now becoming uncontrollable. I say 'thing' because I still didn't know that this 'thing' was depression. I had now reached a tipping point, the point of suicidal ideation. Although football was now over, for a short time at least, my hectic schedule showed no signs of letting up. This was probably the best thing for me given recent events.

Not only had I to contend with the ever-worsening situation going on in my head, but this was also a time of change in my life. This change came in two forms – education and work. Four days before the All Ireland final, I was contacted by Philip Duffy, the manager at Texaco service station, to offer me a job. I went in prior to the final for some training, and was now two weeks into part-time employment.

The job really put me to the pin of my collar right from the start. Naturally enough, as a sales assistant, you're dealing with the public constantly. Regardless of how I was feeling, I had to put up that poker face I'd been so used to over the last two years. Customers were of course unaware of this, especially on the occasions when someone would recognise me as 'Shane, the Dublin footballer'. Why would anyone think I was suicidal, especially just weeks after winning the Sam Maguire at eighteen years of age?

I recall one morning in work, one of my colleagues said, 'Looks like you didn't get much sleep last night.' I blamed a heavy night on the drink, staying up until all hours celebrating with my teammates. This being a few weeks after the All Ireland, it seemed like a plausible explanation. The truth was that I was beginning to have restless nights – constantly tossing and turning as hundreds of thoughts churned around in my head. On occasion, I would break out into tears, leaving my pillow drenched. That had been the case on this morning. I had been awake an hour before I was due to be in work, bed covers wrapped cocoon-like around me and tears streaming down my face, as I asked myself, 'When is this going to get better?'

The two weeks after the final were the most mentally draining ever since depression had come to pay a visit, a little under two years before. My poker face had to be better than ever once I set foot into the workplace. It's a nerve-wrecking time for anyone, starting out in a new job, and I had the added pressure of keeping up the persona that everyone expected of a successful young Dublin footballer.

My first day of college was on the horizon too. Like the transition from primary to secondary school, I just hoped I would fit in with the crowd, and make the transition as seamless as possible.

I remember my first day in Coláiste Dhúlaigh very vividly. I hadn't slept well the night before and, as I sat down to breakfast that morning, I couldn't attach any emotion to the prospect of my first day of college. My mind or body couldn't latch on to anything, it seemed. As I sat into the car to drive to college, a glance in the rear-view mirror showed a pale, expressionless, worn-out figure staring back at me. I had picked out my favourite playlist to play on the way to college, hoping this would help to get me out of the rut I was in. As the journey wore on, my mood lifted ever so slightly. I was fearful of meeting a new group of people for the first time, especially given how I was at this time. But I was somewhat relieved that I could feel again – even if it was fear I was feeling.

Pulling up outside Coláiste Dhúlaigh, I sat in the car for a few moments to regain my composure before heading in. It served little purpose, because I was fidgeting with my clothes, fearful of making eye contact with anyone along the way as I made the short walk from the car park to the building. Once inside, my heart rate spiked again as I attempted to orientate myself. Depression had such a grip on me that the last thing I wanted to do was approach someone to ask where my first class might be. At that moment in my life, this simple task seemed like climbing Mount Everest.

I felt like judging eyes were landing on me as other students buzzed around the corridors, while I stood like a rabbit in headlights. The college wasn't very big, so I decided just to walk and hope that I'd come across my classroom. After probably ten minutes of climbing up and down stairs, passing the same lecture room twice or three times, I stumbled upon the one I was looking for. Walking in, I lifted my head for a millisecond to locate an empty seat, at the very back of the room. Even after I sat down, my head didn't glance to the left or right, such was the paralysing fear that was over me.

This first day was simply an introduction to the modules we'd be taking for the year. As the day came to a close, I hadn't said more than a couple of words to anyone around me. That wasn't in my usual character, and I'm sure I seemed like an arrogant individual to the other students. Even though I was beating myself up inside with how I conducted myself, the prospect of getting to know new people and letting them in scared me to the core.

By November, little had changed in how I was feeling. Although football had taken a back seat over the last month, having a part-time job and college meant I was kept busy. I still kept up some exercise every day, even though it was supposed to be my off season. Inter-county football was starting up again, and now I would be representing the Dublin U21 footballers in my second year at this grade. Almost the entire panel that represented the group the previous year were there again. We had been knocked out very early on in the provincial stages the last time, so now we wanted to make amends. I had begun to question my love for football, and hoped that it would be rekindled with the recommencement of inter-county training. To be honest, I was nervous to find out the outcome.

I didn't have to wait too long. Our first session was in the middle of November, out in Clan na Gael Fontenoy. I knew that my love for the game hadn't wandered too far away, because pretty soon into that first session I felt the 'buzz' that I had been missing.

For the most part, I was settling into college and work. I also had a ten-day trip to Cancun with the entire senior football team to look forward to at the start of December – a reward for winning the All Ireland. How then was I still having suicidal ideations on an almost daily basis? Apart from the brief respite that training continued to give me, my internal life continued to be a living hell. Irrational thoughts constantly passed in and out of my head as I went about my day. I would be waiting to cross the road or standing at a train station, thinking, 'Will I end it all here now?'

Coming into December, with not long left in my first semester in Coláiste Dhúlaigh, my attendance was declining. My parents weren't aware of this at the time. I didn't want to draw attention to myself at home, so I got up every morning around the same time I always did and made my way to college. Or so my parents thought. Instead, I'd drive towards Coolock, stop at the McDonalds drive-through and order an Americano. Then I'd park up, stick my headphones on and either listen to music or watch something on YouTube. I felt more comfortable doing this than attending college. Students in my class were aware of my involvement with the Dublin team at this stage, and they were also aware of the all-expenses-paid trip to Cancun that was coming up. I felt that this put an onus on me now, more than ever, to put up a front like I was this person living the dream life. I was tired of having to put up a front every day.

The same went for my job. I was 'Shane, the footballer', so naturally enough, for customers who had a vague notion of who I was, the first port of call for conversation was about football. It wore me down having to constantly act like everything was wonderful in my world. A number of times over the last few months, I wished I could just not turn up to work, but that would soon have had me fired and questions would then be asked at home.

The trip to Cancun arrived. It was a wet and miserable December morning as management, players, wives, girlfriends and kids gathered in Terminal Two of Dublin Airport, ready to set off for ten days in the sun. It was my first team holiday away, which brought both nerves and excitement. I remember stepping off the plane and being hit by a wave of heat across my face. We arrived at Hotel Riu, home for the next ten days. It was like paradise – all-inclusive hotel, a beach right out back, water activities including banana boating, jet skiing and so on. I roomed with Cormac Costello, a teammate and good friend who had been involved in all the Dublin development squads with me from under-twelves onwards.

For our first day, we were left to settle in and relax after the long day's travel. An itinerary was handed out for the following days of things we might like to do. Structure and routine always served me well to keep my mind distracted when I was back in Ireland, so I got involved in absolutely everything that was on the list – zip-lining, off-roading, golf, snorkelling and all-day boat trips. All of these were absolutely incredible experiences.

There were times on the trip though where we had some down time, and that's when the reality of my situation set in. I'd be sitting on the beach sunbathing, while irrational thoughts passed through my mind. Towards the last few days, I distinctly remember thinking to myself, 'Will this be my last ever Christmas with my family?' Bizarrely, I continued to sit there expressionless, feeling no emotion, as if I was okay with that thought.

The holiday came to an end. As we sat in the airport, preparing to board the plane back home, some of the lads remarked on how they were looking forward to getting home for Christmas and spending some quality time with friends and family. This innocuous remark set me off on a spiral of negative emotions. The thought from a few days previous, 'Will this be my last ever Christmas with my family?' played on repeat in my head for most of the journey home.

I struggled massively in the lead up to Christmas. In work, I constantly wore a fake smile as everyone who came into the shop was in good spirits, with Christmas day fast approaching. Fortunately, football was still going on at this time, so I still had that excuse to pull out of social events with my friends and family. All around me were people content and happy with their lives. 'Why can't I be like that?' I kept asking myself. I honestly felt worthless. There were days when I wanted it all to end. My crutch, my medication, continued to be football – even if it only gave me brief respite from the torment I was feeling more than ever.

I found Christmas Day incredibly challenging. In our house were my parents, my three sisters and their boyfriends. At the breakfast table, I was almost mute for the entire sitting. My mother, as most do, seemed to have a sixth sense for when something wasn't quite right. She asked me, 'Is everything okay?' 'I didn't get much sleep,' I replied. I would later learn that this was the first time my mother sensed something wasn't right with me. I clung on to the excuse of tiredness as I excused myself early from the dinner table that afternoon to go for a nap. I spent the rest of the evening on my own in my room watching a film. I was at the point now where the cracks were harder to hide.

It wasn't only at home that people began to notice something wasn't right. At work, my colleagues were taking notice too. I was coming into work with a pale complexion and bloodshot eyes, having been up for half the night crying. In times gone by, I had placed the blame on a night out on the beer, which was believable as it was my off season. However, now, at the beginning of January and with the pre-season very much underway, that excuse no longer held up. I blamed my appearance on a lack of sleep. I wasn't lying, but because of the regularity of it, I could tell from the looks on my colleagues' faces that they knew it was something deeper.

I didn't know how much longer I'd be able to deal with all of this before doing something irreversible. The lack of sleep, the depressive episodes, the repression of my own identity and the suicidal thoughts – I didn't want to be dealing with it on my own anymore. It shook me to the core, but I began to tell myself that I would have to speak up and tell my parents what was going on. I didn't know what I was going to say, because I couldn't make sense of it in my own head, never mind articulate it to them. The next few weeks was a constant back-and-forth in my head: 'Should I, shouldn't I?' This line of internal dialogue came to a shuddering halt one night in the middle of January.

On Wednesday, 15 January 2014, there was a friendly away match against Cork for the under-21s, as the Championship was fast approaching. My parents would very rarely miss a match, and happily travelled all over the country to support me. On this evening, they did just that. It was a typical January night – bitterly cold, wet and windy. I didn't mind any of that, because I was doing what I loved to do best. I wasn't aware of it at the time, but as we made our way into the dressing room at half time, my mother received a phone call from my uncle Hugh. He gave her the devastating news that my Granddad had passed away. This came as a huge shock, as she had gone to visit him only earlier that day. He had been unwell over the last while, but not to the extent that we thought he was going to pass any time soon.

On the bus home, I was still unaware of what had happened. In fact, on the journey home I was having an internal conversation yet again about opening up to my parents. They arrived home about 11pm, and discussed whether to tell me the news there and then or hold off until the next day. They weren't sure, as I was due to be up at 5.30am for senior training and they didn't want to affect my sleep. They decided that they were going to tell me.

I arrived home just after midnight, dropped my bag in the hall and saw that the light in the kitchen was still on. I went in, to be greeted by my parents and Stephanie, all gathered around the table. I knew straight away that something wasn't quite right. Before I had any time to think, my mother said, 'Shane, unfortunately I got a phone call from Hugh to say that Granddad passed away this evening.' A moment passed as I tried to comprehend what I'd just been told. Such was the pain I was experiencing in my life that I simply wasn't able to attach any emotion to the news. A long moment of silence passed before I said, 'I'm sorry to hear it.' Then I headed out of the kitchen and into my bedroom.

This was a fairly mundane response, to say the least. You'd think by my response that I had little or no relationship with my granddad. In fact, quite the opposite was true. From an early age, I looked up to my granddad. He always took a big interest in anything I was doing in my life. I'd visit him every couple of weeks to fill him in on all that was going on. He was very in tune with everything, and would remember what I had told him on the previous visit. In his later years, he kept up to date with my inter-county career, reading reports on my matches or listening in on the radio, often joking about how I should've scored another ten goals in a certain match!

A few hours after being given the news that Granddad was gone, I was still sitting bolt upright in my bed, unable to attach any sort of emotion to the situation. My parents later admitted they had their suspicions at Christmas that something was up with me, but my reaction to the passing of my granddad certainly gave them reason to be concerned.

The funeral came and went. I told myself that whatever suffering I had been going through couldn't compare to what my mother was going through right then, so I decided to park aside any thoughts of speaking up for the time being. During that time my outlet was sport, not for the first time.

It was now February, a busy period, with the start of the National League with the senior footballers and less than a month until the first round of the under-21 Championship. Some time had now passed since the funeral, and the thought of possibly saying something to my parents came up again. I spent time alone during this period, sometimes going out for a walk or a drive to try to gather my thoughts on what exactly I was going to say to them.

However, the thought of speaking up was to be short-lived again. Only six weeks after the passing of my granddad, my granny passed away too. A feeling of complete and utter devastation crashed through my family – particularly my mam, who in the space of six weeks had now lost both her mother and father. With a protective instinct for my mother, I kept in whatever I was thinking of telling her and my dad for now.

When you're going through times of adversity, very often the smallest of things can mean the most. There were two examples of this on the week of my granny's funeral. The first was when Dessie Farrell, my under-21 manager, came to the burial of my granny. He stood at the back for most of it, but I very much felt his presence there and it meant a great deal.

The second instance was at senior training later in the week. I told Jim Gavin about the passing of my granny. His mantra has always been that 'the person comes before the player', and this rang through when he said, 'If you want some time off training to spend with your family, we'll have no problem with you doing that.' It was something every manager around the country probably would have said, but you just don't know the sort of pressure that players, especially inter-county players, put on themselves to be present and performing at every session. I didn't take any time off. Football was and always will be an outlet for me, and this would especially be the case in the coming month.

The beginning of March saw the start of the under-21 Championship campaign. Our goal was to be crowned All Ireland Champions in May. We were wary, however, of looking too far down the road, having been knocked out in the early stages of the competition by Longford the previous year. Dessie and his management team left no stone unturned in preparing us to face Carlow in the quarter-final of the Leinster Championship.

My mind was elsewhere though in the lead up to the game. In the week of a game, as a player, your mind usually focuses in on the job at hand – who your direct opponent will be and what his strengths and weaknesses are; how the opposing team plays as a whole so that you can plan to exploit any weaknesses. I was too worried about everything that surrounded the game – the pre-match meal, the bus journey to and from the ground and meeting people on the street who would ask about the match.

I think it's hard to truly understand how mentally exhausting it is to put up a front, to pretend everything is okay when it really isn't, unless you've experienced it. The whole week took such a toll on my mind and body that by the time the match came around I was running on fumes. I sat there in the Poitín Stil during our pre-match meal and uttered no more than two words at the table. I don't know whether my teammates sitting at the table just put it down to the passing of my granddad and granny so recently, but they never mentioned anything.

The part I had been worrying about all week was next – the bus journey. Ever since the dark clouds had first descended over me, way back in the middle of fifth year, I never liked going on the team bus. It was the tight, enclosed space, the trapped feeling, that I didn't like. There were also the murmurs you would hear throughout the bus. My irrational mind would go into overdrive here, fearing that my teammates were talking about me and my behaviour. For this journey, I sat up near the front of the bus, put my headphones on and kept my head down. The music distracted me from any irrational thoughts.

We eventually arrived at the ground, and our pre-match routine was underway – a quick walk of the pitch, ten minutes' individual work in the dressing room, pre-match team talk, then out onto the pitch for the warm up. I always felt safe out on the pitch, because I could fully immerse myself in what I loved to do. This game was no different. In the end, we ran out convincing 31-point winners. The bus home had me once again filled with worry, my mind in overdrive. My life was heading in a downward spiral. The constant repression of my own identity meant that the inevitable was only around the corner.

In the days following our Championship game, I began to tell myself once more that I would speak to my parents about what was going on.

Apart from a crippling fear at how they might react, there was also the question of what exactly I would say. The cloudiness was at an all-time high in my head – I simply couldn't hold one thought without hundreds more tumbling in on top of it. I knew I needed to speak up sooner rather than later, because my life was in a mess. By this time, I had stopped attending Coláiste Dhúlaigh completely, though my parents didn't know this, as I was keeping up the act of getting up in the morning and pretending I was going to college. Instead, I continued to sit outside McDonald's in Coolock with my coffee. Here I would contemplate what I might say to my parents.

Football was what I was solely basing my happiness on now – I was on survival mode with anything outside of that. Work did give me brief respite, but I didn't come away from it with the same feeling as I did from football. By now though, I was beginning to get the same associations with training as I did with bus journeys, those feelings of entrapment and paranoia – it was never the training itself but everything that came before and after. It was like this when I sat in the dressing room, having a post-session meal or team meeting.

Our next Championship match was two weeks after our last. In the week leading up to the semi-final against Longford, I made a few conscious changes. I would usually arrive thirty minutes before training, take my time getting changed and do some mobility work before making my way onto the pitch. Now I arrived fifteen minutes before training and already had my training gear on, just leaving me to quickly put my boots on. I now did my mobility work out on the pitch.

I skipped the post-session meals this week too, taking longer in the shower and waiting outside in the fresh air before being called back in for the team meeting. At the team meetings, I sat at the very back – I was paranoid that if I sat up front, people would have an eye on me and notice something wasn't quite right with me. Throughout the entire week, not one of my teammates picked up on anything I was doing differently.

I'm a big believer in sticking to the same routine in the lead up to a match. What I was doing was potentially jeopardising my performance on the pitch, but my whole focused was merely on surviving.

My new match-day routine from before the Carlow game, although not bulletproof, was put into play for the Longford game. For this game, our pre-match meal was in the Louis Fitzgerald hotel and the match was in Portlaoise. As the game got closer, I had concerns over the potential collapse of my performance due to the week I had had, but my concerns were quickly put to rest once the ball was thrown up. I was able to fully immerse myself in the game, and I put in a good performance. We came out on top by ten points, booking ourselves a spot in the Leinster final against age-old rivals Meath. The following few weeks would be my most defining yet.

I felt like I was imprisoning the person I wanted to be. I kept thinking back to times in my life when crippling depression wasn't in control of my life. I desperately wished that I could go back to being that person, but I didn't know how to get in contact with him again.

I reached my lowest point just days after the semi-final against Longford. The suicidal ideations I was having for many months now were gaining more of my attention. My avoidance of nearly everything wasn't helping. I made up every sort of excuse not to meet up with my friends. This meant that I left myself isolated and vulnerable at home, ruminating for hours at a time. It was here, during these times, that I began to think more and more about dying by suicide. It sounds bizarre, but I found a sort of comfort when these thoughts were running through my head.

I'm ashamed to admit it, but never once around this time did I think of the impact it would have on my family, friends, teammates and further afield. The only thing I was thinking was, 'I've found a solution to my problem.' At more rational times, it frightened me, to say the least, that I was becoming more and more comfortable with the thought of dying by suicide. My time was almost up, I felt. That was until the morning of the Leinster final, when the process of rebuilding my life began.

CHAPTER 4

THOSE TWO WEEKS

Wednesday, 2 April, was the morning of the Leinster final. I was sitting on the edge of the couch in the sitting room with my hood up, hunched over with my head in my hands. On the floor, between my legs, was a flood of tears. I could hear my mother, the only other person in the house at the time, make her way down the stairs and into the kitchen. She called in to me, 'Do you want breakfast?' I wiped away the tears that were streaming down my face, cleared my throat and replied 'yes, please.' I hadn't yet sat my parents down – I was still covering up the fact that there was anything wrong, but they had known for some time that I hadn't been right. Since Christmas time, the passing of my granny and granddad, the bloodshot eyes, my gradual avoidance of most things, there were all sorts of signs that something was up.

This was why my mother was still in the house. As she entered the sitting room with my bowl of porridge that apparently I couldn't make for myself at nineteen years of age, I didn't have it in me to cover it up anymore. I didn't even peer up to acknowledge her presence in the room. I stayed bowed down, in what seemed a never-ending stream of tears. She took a seat beside me, put her arm around my shoulder and stayed silent for a moment. Then she said, 'It's okay, Shane, we're all here for you. You can tell us anything.' I said nothing.

Internally, I was frustrated. I couldn't make sense of all the noise going on in my head, never mind articulate it to my mother. I'm sure she was feeling frustrated too, wanting to help but without enough information to know what to do. Eventually, as the tears dried, I began to shed a bit of light on the situation. I didn't say a whole lot, because the cloudiness in my head wouldn't allow me to. I did, however, tell her I had been feeling that way for some time, and that recently I had had thoughts of dying by suicide. I didn't feel any immediate relief after saying this. If anything, I felt guilty for burdening my mother with it. Nevertheless, the first small step in laying the foundation to rebuild my life had been taken.

My mum knew she needed to get me out of the house, at least for a few hours, to distract me before the game that evening. She contacted my middle sister, Mairead, who was off work that day too. I went upstairs to get ready and waited for her to arrive – I didn't know where she would be bringing me. She arrived a short time later and off in the car we went.

Even though Mairead knew I had been crying for most of the morning, I still tried to hide my tears. It didn't last long though – soon after entering the car, I was in a flood of tears yet again, with no explanation why. My whole life was dark. I wanted to be put out of the pain of it all. My mind was going from these dark thoughts back to the car and the sound of Mairead's voice. I wasn't responding to anything she said, but I found a certain comfort in the sound of her voice.

We arrived at the destination Mairead had chosen, Howth cliff walk. Why she chose to go on a cliff walk on the afternoon of a Leinster final, I'll never know! Howth cliff walk is well known for the picturesque views it offers, but my gaze hardly left the ground. I didn't speak more than five words the entire way around, though I knew I had a listening ear right beside me should I choose to speak up. It felt like a short break from the inner demons, but before I knew it we were back at the car. It was as if the moment I shut the car door, my nightmare began again. Hundreds of thoughts raced through my mind, but none stayed long enough for me to grasp onto.

This was the first time I considered that not even football could do anything for me. I told my sister I was going to contact Dessie and tell him I was unavailable for the match. 'If that's what will make this easier for you, do it,' she said. I took out my phone and scrolled down to his name in my phonebook. I stared at the phone for a moment, my heart racing. 'What will I say?' I asked myself. A few moments passed, as I stared at his name on my screen. I was trying to conjure up an excuse, doubt spinning in my head at every thought that came to me. I locked the phone and put it back in my pocket. Mairead stared over at me, but said nothing. I don't know, still to this day, why I didn't follow through with that phone call.

We arrived back home a short while later. Little was said, and my parents didn't question whether I was going to play the match or not. They left me to pack my bag in peace. All the while, my stomach was churning. I was almost at the point of getting sick, I was so nervous. I feared how I would be for the pre-match meal, for the bus journey and then not to mention the match itself, which would be played in front of thousands of fans. As my Dad dropped Scooby and myself to the Louis Fitzgerald hotel, I was still unsure whether I would go ahead and play.

There was a lot going on in the room where we met up. Our physio, Cillian, was in one corner, doing strapping for players; others were doing foam rolling and mobility in another corner; management were talking to individual players; and between all of that, there was the pre-match meal too. I kept busy with three out of the four things happening in the room. The one I didn't entertain was the pre-match meal, which I didn't feel I could stomach – hardly the ideal preparation for a Leinster final.

I took up my customary seat at the front of the bus as we set off for Portlaoise. 'I can't go through with this, I can't, I can't,' I said to myself. I turned the volume all the way up on my headphones, desperately hoping that the sound of the music would drown out the negative voices in my head. I had carefully chosen my playlist, full of songs that brought me back to happy moments in my life. It served me well for the first part of the journey, but soon the negative voices began to speak louder. I sent Mairead a text, saying, 'I really don't think I can play.' Almost immediately, she replied, saying, 'You can. Stay up the front of the bus and put that poker face on.' I turned up the volume on my headphones once more, shut my eyes so hard that my face began to wince and paid attention to every lyric that was being played in my head.

After what seemed a lifetime, we arrived at the ground. We made our way up the long corridor; halfway up was our dressing room. By this time, I had decided I was going to play. I didn't go out to walk the pitch; instead, I got changed and eagerly awaited the start of the game. As my teammates came back in from the pitch to get changed, key messages were read out by the management. Very little of what they said was registering with me. I just sat, visualising the ball being thrown up for the start of the game.

The warm up took place on a training pitch just behind the stadium. This meant my family were still unsure whether I would play any part in the game. After the warm up came Dessie's final words back in the dressing room. One of my superstitions during this year was that I had to be the last player out on the pitch. My parents were left to wonder, right up until the very last player emerged from the tunnel, whether I would play. We lined up for 'Amhrán na bhFiann', and then the ball was thrown up.

The following sixty minutes was, still to this day, the most satisfying I have ever played. I was like a kid again, chasing every ball and simply getting immersed in it all. I think that when I was out there, I was very literally running away from my problems. With the frantic nature of the game, I'd say most players were glad to hear the half-time whistle. However, it was an inconvenience to me; I didn't want half time to come. When it did though, we found ourselves four points up.

The ball was thrown up for the second half, and I was back to where I had left off, pounding every blade of grass, wishing it would last forever. I would have stayed out there all night if I could. I distinctly remember peering over at the referee near the end of the game, wanting him to keep it going. We were five points up – I should have been willing him to blow it up!

A goalmouth scramble in the dying seconds meant we were all in close proximity as the final whistle blew. It's difficult to take a moment like this in, as you're congratulating any blue jersey that comes up to you for an embrace. In the midst of all of it, John Costello, Dublin County Board Chief Executive, came up and told me I'd been awarded Man of the Match. It all happened very quickly – before I knew it, I was walking up the steps to receive my award.

Here I was again, on a pedestal, receiving an award, getting a huge round of applause from the travelling supporters. I couldn't help but think of where I had been twelve hours previously, as my mother found me in a flood of tears. Little did these supporters know the inner turmoil I'd been experiencing for over two years now.

After the presentation, I was ushered down to the tunnel to do short interviews for newspapers and radio stations. I uttered the usual soundbite answers that players give after a win. Then I joined the rest of the players in the dressing room. Naturally, celebrations were taking place, but I took no part in them. All I wanted to do was shower up and get home. I quickly got changed as my teammates continued to celebrate around me.

I made my way out toward Dessie, who was standing at the dressing room door. I took him aside and told him I was going home with my parents, who were waiting outside the ground. I also told him I was going to Sweden the next day to visit my sister, Michelle, for a couple of days. This trip was booked only a couple of weeks ago. Although my parents didn't say it to me at the time, their hope was that whatever I was perceived to be holding in, I'd confide in my sister.

The All Ireland semi-final was in two and a half weeks, and Dessie didn't have an issue with me heading away for a few days. 'That's fine. Is everything okay, Shane?' he said. I knew by the way he asked the question that he could sense something was a little off. 'Yeah, of course, I'm just shattered after the game,' I said. I knew he didn't believe me, but he let me on my way.

The next morning, I woke up feeling numb. Neither the Leinster title nor the Man of the Match award gave me any satisfaction. The prospect of a few days away in Stockholm to visit my sister also did nothing to lift my mood. My dad dropped me out to the airport in the afternoon. Along the way, he said, 'Whatever it is, don't be afraid to have a conversation with Michelle at some point. We're all here to help.' 'I will,' I said.

Internally, I was frustrated. My parents placed great hope in this trip.

I've always confided in Michelle a bit more than in anyone else in the family. However, what I was dealing with was on a much larger scale than any problem I'd come to her with before. As I stood in line to board the plane to Stockholm, I began to visualise the conversation I'd have with my sister. Throughout the flight, I searched desperately for reasoning behind my inner turmoil, but nothing was making sense for me.

I had three days to spend with my sister. This may sound like sufficient time to open up a conversation about what was going on – I thought so prior to the trip. However, when I was faced with the reality of the situation, everything changed. My sister made it clear on my first day over there that she wasn't going to push me for answers. 'Whenever you feel like talking, I'm here,' she said. The fact was, however, that I didn't have anything more to share than what I had already told my parents. I've always confided in my sister, but this was different. If anything, I was finding it harder to share anything at all with her. How could I tell my sister, who lives thousands of miles away, that her little brother no longer wanted any part of this world?

On my first night there, I decided to tell her everything – everything I had already told my parents. The reason for this decision was the thoughts I was having while lying restlessly in bed. The noises in my head that were keeping me up until the early hours were giving me a way out. My irrational mind was telling me to die by suicide over here in Stockholm. 'That way it'll be easier for my family and friends at home,' I told myself. This was clearly an absurd thought process to have, but such was the power my irrational mind had at this point. On the occasions when I went from irrational to rational thoughts, I knew I had to speak up. I was becoming fearful that I would begin to rationalise the thought of dying by suicide, and then act on it.

The following day, we planned to go for brunch along Torsgatan, a street well known for its cafés. Michelle and my brother in law, Joey, were doing most of the talking on the ten-minute walk. I was switching from internal to external voices every few seconds, like flicking between two radio stations. As we neared the café, my mind was focused on the internal dialogue. I was playing out various scenarios as to how my sister would react to what I was about to tell her. My heart was beating fast, and my hands were moving frantically too – they were in my pockets, then scratching my head, then fixing my clothes, over and over. I could feel Michelle and Joey peering over out of the corners of their eyes.

Without saying anything, I veered towards a wall and sat down. I leaned over, elbows on my knees and hands on my head, and began crying. Michelle and Joey sat on either side of me and comforted me. We were sitting on a very busy street, with passersby looking on I'm sure, but my emotional cap had been lifted and the outpouring of pain was uncontrollable. I just wished that it would end soon.

After perhaps ten minutes, the well ran dry. I sat upright, wiping the remaining tears away. 'I don't want to feel like this anymore,' I said. A short pause. 'I don't think I can do this,' I muttered. 'What's going on for you, Shane? We can help if you tell us what's going on,' Michelle said. Hearing the hurt in Michelle's voice made it all the more difficult. I was desperate though. My second cry for help was on the way. 'I don't know, Michelle. It's been going on for two years now. I don't think I can deal with it for much longer. I don't want to be here anymore,' I said with a lump in my throat, trying to hold back the tears again.

Michelle and Joey are by no means psychologists, but their actions following this allowed me to open a door I never even knew existed. They stayed silent, and Michelle simply placed a comforting hand on my back, almost like a silent acknowledgement of what I had told her. Like a few days before, along the Howth cliff walk with Mairead, I felt I had a listening ear beside me. The difference was that I used the listening ear on this day. Having not been judged on my first outpouring, I opened up a bit more, albeit slightly hesitantly. I spoke about how I regularly put on a poker face in school. I shared snippets of information every few minutes, each time waiting for the judgement to come, but it never did. I'd be lying if I said the clouds that were hanging over me all this time were gone, but after an hour of sharing how I felt, the sky became that bit clearer.

Over the next few days, I continued to share some of my experiences from the past two years with Michelle and Joey. Although I had now added a very useful coping mechanism to what I would later call my 'mental health toolbox', I was still short of some tools. Yes, talking about my emotions helped. Yes, physical exercise helped. And yes, music helped. However, there is only so much you can get out of them in any one day. In the times when I wasn't utilising one of these three, I was left to do battle with the never-ending negative dialogue in my head. Michelle recalled, 'As the days wore on, although you were speaking up, we could see from your face that you cut an exhausted figure.'

Michelle and Joey organised a meal out for my last night in Stockholm, in a restaurant called Restaurang AG – a steakhouse regularly rated as the best in Stockholm. We were all sitting at the table, our main course about to be served. I had hardly spoken a word up to this point, nor managed even to fake a smile – I was physically drained. As my sixteen-ounce sirloin steak was placed on the table, Michelle was beaming from ear to ear, probably thinking, 'If there's anything in the world that will bring a smile to his face, it's what has just been placed in front of him.' But the expression on my face didn't change. My mind was elsewhere – glum, motionless, defeated.

I was dreading going back to Ireland. Ireland itself wasn't the cause of my decline over the last two years. The dread I felt about going back was more to do with associating so many negative memories with places I so often visited. This was a topic of conversation I brought up with Michelle and Joey during my stay. I didn't need to tell them I wasn't ready to go home – it was written all over my face. Toward the end of the meal, Michelle asked, 'How would you feel about staying for a bit longer, Shane? Joey is flying out to Copenhagen tomorrow for two days on a business trip. If you wanted, you could join him.' Without a moment's hesitation, I said, 'Yes.'

Back at the apartment, we booked the flights. I would now go to Copenhagen until Wednesday night, then fly back to Stockholm and stay a further four days. I would fly back to Ireland on the Sunday, almost a full week later than originally planned. I had the small matter of an All Ireland semi-final in two weeks – this wouldn't be the ideal preparation for it. Michelle helped me that evening to compose an email to Dessie. It included my plans for the next six days, and assured him I'd be keeping on top of my fitness while over here. If his suspicions regarding my wellbeing on the night of the Leinster final weren't aroused, then this email would certainly get him wondering. Then I signed out of my emails. I wasn't made aware of it at the time, but for the remainder of my stay abroad, Dessie and my parents were in constant contact regarding my wellbeing. Also unknown to me, Dessie had made an appointment for me to see a psychologist for the Wednesday following my arrival home. However, through a series of unforeseen circumstances, this never materialised.

I was very much looking forward to spending a few days in Copenhagen. There were terms and conditions to abide by for the course of my stay, however: Because Joey was going there on a business trip, he would be away from me for most of each day. This thought scared my mother to the core – so much so that she considered flying over to meet us in Copenhagen, to be by my side when Joey wasn't. Instead of this, we agreed that I would be in contact with at least one person from my family every hour.

I stayed in contact with my mother the majority of the time. On occasion, I'd speak to Michelle, Stephanie or Mairead. Of course, I spoke to Joey too. In between these conversations, I went back to what served me well in Ireland. I created a structure to my day. I made good use of the gym facilities at the hotel, using it twice a day. I set targets for this each day – a target for each of my morning and afternoon sessions, which were split into cardio and weight-based work. I was not only eliciting the natural 'feel-good' benefits that come from a bout of exercise – setting targets also allowed my mind to fixate on these, rather than the irrational thoughts.

When I completed my afternoon session, I would take a walk into the city centre. I always had my headphones on along the way, playing a selection of songs that brought me back to happier times in my life. I'd sit down at a coffee shop, waiting for Joey to finish his work. He would meet me and we would walk around the city, searching for places to go for dinner each evening.

I found myself drained at the end of each day. This was due to the fast-paced way I was living my life at this time – I needed to be doing something from the minute I woke up to the minute my head hit the pillow. That's how I coped. I managed to stay afloat until Wednesday, when the trip to Copenhagen came to an end. Really though, I wasn't living anymore, I was just surviving.

My remaining four days in Stockholm were filled with worry and despair. My appreciation for life had hit an all-time low. As each day passed, I retreated further and further into my shell. Michelle and Joey tried their level best to keep my mind occupied and positive, bringing me out to parks, sightseeing in the city, going to cafés and restaurants. At this stage I was mute. The only conversation going on was the one in my head. My mind was being overrun with negative judgements and thoughts about myself. 'Things aren't going to get better for you,' I told myself, and really, what evidence did I have over the past while to suggest that this wasn't true?

On my final night in Stockholm, we ordered a takeaway and planned to sit in for the evening. I had other ideas, however. The previous September had been the first time I had thoughts of dying by suicide. Since then, it had never been too far from my thoughts. I never wanted to act out what I was thinking, but nonetheless it was a thought that paid a visit way too often. Since the turn of the year, the thought of dying by suicide was becoming louder and louder. I was hoping that now that my family were aware of my situation, they would give me the answers I didn't have. How could they though? They aren't qualified doctors or psychologists. They were doing everything in their power to help me, with the little information they had. 'If my family haven't got the answers, then what would a doctor or psychologist know?' I asked myself, and this led back to the irrational thought that I didn't want to be part of this world anymore.

While Michelle and Joey sat watching television, I got up and put on my jacket and shoes. 'I'm going out for a walk. I'll be back in a while,' I told them. 'Okay. Don't be long,' Michelle replied, worry etched all over her face. I made my way down the spiral staircase of Michelle and Joey's apartment as the thought crossed my mind: 'Will that be the last time I see them?' I wasn't going out intending to die by suicide, but such thoughts were coming into my mind regularly by now. I was going out in an attempt to mute the inner demons that were talking far too loudly and too often on this day.

I was out in the cold of the night with my hood up, headphones on and a desperate wish that things were going to get better. I didn't walk too far. In fact, I sat down on a park bench only five hundred metres away from the apartment. Soon I found myself in an all-too-familiar position – bent over with my elbows on my knees and head in my hands, crying. I searched desperately for the smallest sensation of happiness to pass through my body. It wasn't coming though.

I felt I had come to the end of my road, and this feeling left me paralysed. I visualised many ways I could die by suicide, there and then, on this potentially fateful night. I broke down crying at the horrific images that were passing through my mind. I recall compressing my hands on either side of my head, as if trying to crush the crippling thoughts that were going on inside. 'Stop, stop, stop!' the voice in my head was saying.

I reached into my pocket for my phone. Hands trembling, I sent a text to one of my best friends, Moe. It simply read, 'Can you talk?' His response was instant: 'Yeah, everything alright?' I took a few deep breaths before pressing the call button. Moe answered straight away. 'Hello,' he said. I tried to respond, but I was all choked up. Eventually I came back with, 'Moe, I need to tell …' Tears streamed down my face before I could finish what I wanted to say. Moe, presumably confused at where this conversation was going, remained calm and waited for me to regain my composure.

What followed was a conversation I'm sure Moe never expected to have. I let him in on what my life had really been like for the past two years. He was clearly shocked by what I was revealing to him. He was a figure in the stories I was sharing with him – he simply hadn't seen beyond the mask I wore so well.

I was drip-feeding Moe these stories, as I was unable to hold myself together for more than a few minutes at a time. I felt like I was reliving all the horrible events as I was describing them. I reached a point where the pain I was reliving became too much, and I blurted out, 'I can't do this anymore, Moe.' I broke down into tears yet again. Moe didn't have to guess what I meant by this statement. To this day, I tell him that the conversation that ensued from here saved my life that night.

Moe and I were never meant to be best friends – we were completely different to each other. That was until we formed a bond that no one could break, on our second year school trip to Germany. We shared a room with two others from our class, but Moe and I were awake until all hours of the night, talking about anything and everything. From here, we went on to become best friends.

He reminded me of this exact moment on the phone as he tried to haul me back to happier moments in my life. He summoned up many other times in the past, when I was living life to the full, assuring me that those days would return again. He painted these pictures so vividly for me, allowing me to escape from the inner turmoil I'd been experiencing. I knew that I wanted to go back to how my life had once been, but too often the cloudiness in my head wouldn't allow me to do this. However, Moe managed to clear some of that for me during this phone call.

Once he had gotten the sense that he had brought me back to reality, he asked if I would make my way back to Michelle and Joey. I thanked him before getting off the phone and returning to the apartment, three hours after I had left. Michelle embraced me as I stood at the kitchen sink, drinking a glass of water. I would later learn that Joey was meanwhile scouring the streets of Stockholm, worried sick that I'd done something irreversible. Thankfully, I hadn't.

The next morning, I woke up with what felt like a ten-stone jacket on me. I was filled with dread. The flight I was due to catch that afternoon played a major part in this feeling. I had been running away from what was inevitable – my return home to Dublin. Although I had managed to get a few more things off my chest than maybe I would have at home, my situation hadn't improved all that much. My major concern in going home was that I would be back in places and situations that I had already formulated negative perceptions of. I didn't know if I could handle facing them anymore. However, the time had come and I had no choice but to return home.

I reluctantly packed my bag, tears streaming down my face at the thought of it all. In times past I would have said my goodbyes at Michelle and Joey's apartment, walked for ten minutes into the city and caught the Arlanda Express train, which takes you directly to the airport. However, such was my reluctance to travel home that Michelle and Joey decided to come along to the airport to make sure I got onto the flight. For the entire journey to the airport, I kept my head bowed, wiping away the tears. The sheer volume of tears meant my eyesight was becoming blurred, much like my thought process.

We reached the airport, and stood for a few moments as I wiped away the remaining tears. I lifted my head to focus my tear-soaked, bloodshot eyes on Michelle and Joey. I wept once more as I embraced them both. 'Will you promise me you'll get on that flight?' Michelle said. I didn't care to clear the lump in my throat; instead, I nodded to acknowledge what she had said. I turned and made my way through the front doors of the airport.

I had arrived slightly ahead of time for my flight. After going through the usual rigmarole of passport check and security check, I headed to the departure gate. I could sense the panic reverberating from my family, because before I could even settle into my seat at the departure gate, I received a number of texts from both Michelle and my parents, looking for updates on where I was. It probably sounds like the most normal and mundane thing to do – to send a text – but when you're going through a time like this, it is easy to lose touch with reality and forget that there are people out there who love and care for you.

That's exactly what these texts did for me – they kept me in touch with reality. Prior to receiving the messages, part of my mind was telling me that if I didn't get on the flight, nobody would even notice. Not for the first time, a completely absurd, irrational thought was solidifying in my mind. However, these small acts of love and care by my family allowed me to keep a hold of reality, even if it was by a fingertip.

Before joining the queue to board the flight, I peered down at my blank phone screen, embarrassed by my reflection. I barely made eye contact with the flight attendant as I handed over my boarding ticket. The flight was only half full, so we had a choice of seats. I chose a seat at the very back of the plane, five rows from the next nearest passenger.

For the next two hours, it was me, my music and my irrational thoughts. With my music playing at full volume, I tried to latch on to happier thoughts and memories. However, only thirty minutes into the flight, I took my familiar posture yet again – leaning over with my elbows on my knees and hands on my head, crying. I could feel the air hostesses' eyes fixing on me as they passed through the aisle. I couldn't control what seemed a never-ending stream of tears. I tried to figure out why I was crying, but the cloudiness in my head wouldn't allow me to. I felt a tap on my shoulder, and I barely brought my eyes up to waist height as a bottle of water and some tissues were put in front of me. I managed to raise my head for a second to acknowledge the gesture.

My sister Mairead and brother in law Colin were waiting at arrivals in Dublin for me. I spoke only a few words on the way home. My suicidal ideations were accelerating at this point, pulling me further and further away from reality. I did, however, cling on to some sense of reality, and that reality led me to text Dessie. Dessie had previous with depression and he was also formerly a psychiatric nurse. Maybe he could give me the answers I simply didn't have? I asked whether we could meet the following day for a coffee and a chat. He responded almost immediately, 'Yes, of course. I'll meet you in Costa coffee in Santry for 10am, Shane.'

That evening, my mother, my sisters Mairead and Stephanie and I went out for a meal. Although they didn't say it, I knew the intention behind this was to keep me distracted. I remember very little of this meal, such was my detachment from reality. My mother later recalled a memory from that evening. She noted how pale I was, and how I became restless at the table, making numerous trips to the toilet. When a question was asked, I peered up glassy-eyed and gave one- or two-word answers. There were moments when I would come out of the trance I was in, but I couldn't engage in conversation for any length of time.

The meal came to an end. It was getting late, approaching 10.30pm, as we made our way home. My mother, Mairead and Stephanie went into the kitchen, while I went up to my bedroom for a few moments, before deciding I wanted to mute the voices in my head by going for a drive. I got the car keys from the hall, told my family I was going out for a drive, and made a sharp exit.

Driving along to my favourite music had worked for me in the past. However, the inner demons had too much of a stranglehold on me at this point, and the suicidal ideations were speaking loud and clear. I've regularly driven out to Howth and that's where I found myself heading for. The playlist that I had on, although loud, may as well not have been playing. The inner demons were getting louder and louder.

I parked up at Howth summit, turned the engine off and lowered the music. 'I won't have to put up with this anymore if I end it all here and now,' I said internally. Looking back, the frightening thing was that this thought gave me a feeling of calm. I'm ashamed to admit it, but I didn't give one thought to my family or friends while this harrowing thought was trying to make itself a reality.

My attention was drawn to the cup holder in the car, where my phone was. The bright light coming up out of the phone was a text message. The message was from Mairead, and it read, 'Hey, think about heading home soon. Mam is worried sick. We love you very much x.' This text awakened my rational mind. 'There are people who care for you,' I thought. Before my irrational mind could reply, I hurriedly turned the engine on and headed home. I don't know whether I was going to follow through with what I was thinking that night, but my sister's message allowed me to remain afloat a little while longer.

The following morning, I was set to meet Dessie in Costa coffee in Santry. My dad decided to bring me over to meet him. My guess is that he was worried about me driving alone – and I don't blame him! On the short journey over, my Dad unintentionally served as a very much needed distraction mechanism. Unsurprisingly, the topic of conversation was sport. I think he knew that this was something I'd engage in. Being avid

Manchester United supporters, we spoke about the game that had been played at the weekend. We moved on to discussing my next game, the All Ireland semi-final versus Cavan in less than one weeks' time.

As we approached Santry, my engagement in the conversation became less and less. I switched to the internal dialogue in my head, wondering, 'What will I say to Dessie?' We arrived at the crowded café. It took a moment to pick out Dessie, sitting in the far left-hand corner. I took my seat and we engaged in small talk to start off with. The dreaded question soon came though: 'So tell me, what's going on?' This triggered my mind to spin into overdrive. I was trying to filter through hundreds of thoughts, attempting to pick out one thing to share with him. Thoughts were coming in quicker than I was able to recognise them for what they were, only adding to the cloudiness.

Such was my inability to control my emotions, I began crying. The poker face that I had worn so proudly for the past two years was well and truly done with. People were all around, having their morning coffee, and here was I, a six-foot-three-inch young man, in a flood of tears amongst it all. I was embarrassed, but I couldn't do anything to control the flow of tears. 'It's okay, Shane. Take a minute there, you'll be fine,' Dessie said.

Between bouts of tears, I filled Dessie in on what had been happening inside me over the last two years, and the point it had gotten to where I had considered dying by suicide in recent months. He confided with me and shared personal experiences of his own, resonating very much with things I had gone through. This was the first time I had heard someone else describe similar experiences. I'm not saying that in that instant I immediately felt better, but I did find comfort in hearing that I wasn't the only one who'd gone such turmoil.

We sat there for just under an hour. Dessie finished off by promising he'd get the help I deeply needed. He would organise an appointment with a psychologist in a few days' time. 'I promise you it'll get better from here,' Dessie said, putting his arm across my shoulder as I exited the coffee shop, my head bowed still, filled with embarrassment. I sat into the car while my dad and Dessie spoke. My dad returned to the car minutes later, patting me on the head and saying, 'That's the first step over and done with. I'm proud of you, son.'

The following morning I was in work. I was awake for the majority of the night with my mind racing, which didn't make the 6am start in work any easier. I was mentally and physically drained from all that had gone on in the last number of weeks. My colleague Tanya remarked, 'You look shattered, Shane. Did you get much sleep last night?' 'No, I was up late watching television,' I told her.

I was only in for a four-hour shift, as we had a training camp in DCU with the U21s. My mother was in constant contact over the four hours. I told her how I was feeling, and she got my dad to drop down with medication to ease the nausea I was experiencing. My dad told me he would bring me to training also. My mind then switched to worrying about facing up to the lads, having been away since the Leinster final.

My four hour shift came to an end. I dropped the car home, got my gear bag, and my dad and I were on our way to DCU. Like the day before, my dad did most of the talking. Training wasn't due to start until 11am. When we were about five minutes away from the pitch, I glanced to the clock on my dad's dash. It read 10:25am. I swiftly cut across my dad mid-sentence, to ask whether we could pull up in Na Fianna GAA club on Mobhi Road – a stone's throw away from the DCU pitches. My Dad didn't question this strange request; he simply answered, 'No problem.' There was a moment's silence then, that I thought I needed to fill. I quite quickly and anxiously said, 'I don't want to arrive too early, because I'll be sat in the dressing room for too long.' 'That's okay,' my Dad said, as we pulled into the Na Fianna car park.

I couldn't sit still, rubbing my hands up and down my thighs and rocking back and forth. A crippling fear came over me and once again, hundreds of thoughts ran through my mind, too many to make sense of. My emotional tap was opened too, and tears streaming down my pale, worried face. My dad comforted me, patting me on the back. 'It's okay, get it all out there,' he said.

Shortly before training was due to start, I wiped away the remaining tears before my dad steered us around to DCU St Clare's. Although I had shown vulnerability in front of my dad, it was the last thing I was going to do in front of my teammates. My dad knew this too. 'Head up, you'll be fine when you get on that pitch, son,' he said. I took a long, deep breath before I opened the car door, and headed for the dressing room.

The first person I met was Philip McElwee, a selector on Dessie's management team. 'Welcome back!' he said with a wry smile – a smile that is so synonymous with him. I continued on to the dressing room. Sure enough, good-natured jeers sprang up from various corners of the room. 'Ah, Carthy, you decided to come back!' I managed to crack a smile in response.

I got my gear on in record time and ran out onto the pitch, conversing very little along the way. As I crossed the white line onto the pitch, my troubles were placed there and forgotten about for the duration of the session. It was me, an open field and footballs; it was heaven! I didn't want the session to end. When it did, my troubles that I had placed on the side of the pitch were waiting for me. Everything got very dark, very quickly.

The next thing on the agenda was a meeting due to take place in the Castleknock hotel, just twenty minutes away from DCU. I hurriedly made my way back to the dressing room to shower up. The atmosphere around me in the dressing room was relaxed, but it was anything but that internally. I fumbled in my bag for my towel and change of clothes, avoiding making eye contact with anyone around me for fear of a conversation being struck up. My heart was beating at a rate I had never experienced before.

I hadn't even fully dried myself when I made a quick exit out to the car park where my Dad was waiting. I got into the car. 'Is everything okay?' Dad asked. 'Can you just drive please?' I replied, struggling to control my breathing. As was the case for much of the previous two years, I didn't know what was causing such a sense of panic. It felt like with each passing minute in the car, the volume of the inner demons was getting louder and louder.

We reached Castleknock village before it all got too much for me, and I asked my dad to pull over to the side of the road. He pulled into a pub car park. What transpired next was a panic attack, and the event was recalled by my Dad, Dessie and Mick Galvin – I have no real memory of it. I got out of the car and walked gingerly over to a wall about ten metres away. Placing my hand on the wall, slightly hunched over, I tried desperately to regain my breath, but I was unable to do so. I went back over to the car, dropped to my knees by the back left wheel and began slamming my hands against my head as if trying to fend off the voices that were on full volume. 'Stop! Stop! My head! My head!' I shouted repeatedly.

My Dad came to my side in an attempt to stem the flow of my panic attack. My screams only grew louder. I began vomiting, such was the stress my body was under. I peered up at one stage, staring down the barrel of my dad's eyes, but as he recalls, 'You had a glass-eyed look that struggled to acknowledge any human existence in front of you.' He rang Dessie, who was already at Castleknock hotel. He advised my Dad to head there, and he did so.

We arrived at the hotel, where Dessie and Mick were waiting. Dessie opened the passenger door, where I was sitting, head in my hands, curled over in an almost fetal position. I eventually sat up, with Dessie patting the back of my head. He asked if I'd like to go for a walk. 'Okay,' I answered. We slowly made our way through the car park toward the golf course. I can't recall what was said, but I know that Dessie was doing all the talking.

Meanwhile, back at the car, Mick was making phone calls to try to get me into St Patrick's mental hospital. We would need a letter from our local GP in Portmarnock before we could go to the hospital. Mick rang the GP to notify him of our imminent arrival. Then Mick gestured to Dessie that it was time to go. As we walked back to the car, Dessie explained to me where I'd be going and that I'd be in the best hands possible. I was still absent from reality, only vaguely aware of what he was telling me.

The team meeting at the hotel was still going ahead. Dessie, being the manager, had to be there, so he couldn't come with me. He embraced me and promised he'd be back with me later on. We got into the car and my dad, Mick and myself were on our way to the GP. Mick recalls that I had calmed down from the earlier hysterics I was in, and was now sitting silently, staring at the dashboard in front of me. I clearly hadn't regained any sense of reality at this point.

In Portmarnock, the doctor briefly assessed me. I was still incoherent at this point, so my dad and Mick filled him in on the recent events. Soon we were on our way to the hospital with the letter of referral. Mick rang ahead to let them know I was coming.

We were met at the hospital by three therapists, who gave me attention immediately. By this point, I had begun to come around. I began to communicate again, but without much clarity. We were shown into a meeting room, where my dad, Mick and I sat down for an initial assessment. Questions were directed at my dad and Mick, mostly dealing with the events that had transpired throughout that day. The meeting lasted about thirty minutes. We then awaited the call from the secondary psychologist, who would be speaking to me directly. We were sitting in the waiting area when Dessie arrived. He embraced me, saying, 'You look a lot better than earlier on.' I was coming around more, and even began engaging in the conversation that was going on between the three lads.

Soon, I was called into the meeting room on my own to discuss things further with the psychologist. I spent a little under an hour with him, trying to build a picture of what had happened over the past two years. The cloudiness in my head was at an all-time high, and I found it difficult to articulate past events. The psychologist felt that I had had enough for one sitting, and he was right, I was exhausted! I came out of the meeting in something of a daze. I sat back down at the table with the three lads as we were told to wait a little while as they got a room ready for me.

Everything that had happened that day still hadn't quite registered with me – the panic attack in the pub car park, the journey to the GP and then to St Patrick's mental hospital, and finally the meetings with two psychologists. I tried to comprehend it, becoming visibly overwhelmed by the thought of it all. Dessie recognised this, and took me outside to get some fresh air. The realisation of where I was was slowly registering with me.

Dessie described what the next twenty-four hours would look like for me. I couldn't quite comprehend what he was saying, breaking down into tears once more and embracing him. 'You're in the right place, Shane. This is the start of your journey to recovery,' he said.

Soon we were notified that my room was ready. Dessie and Mick said their goodbyes. The nurse on shift showed my dad and I to my room, in the Dean Swift Ward – a semi-secure unit where I would begin my journey to recovery. The nurse made sure I was okay for everything, offering me food and water, which I declined.

My Dad and I took a few minutes to say goodbye. He reiterated what Dessie had said to me outside, adding he'd be back up early in the morning with my mam. We shared one more embrace before he went on his way. I lay my head on the pillow and it didn't take long before I was asleep. The following morning would mark my most difficult challenge in life to date.

CHAPTER 5

ELEVEN WEEKS THAT CHANGED MY LIFE

Wednesday, 16 April 2014. I was woken up by two softly spoken nurses, standing at either side of my bed. 'Good morning, Shane,' they said. I was still a bit dazed, having just woken up, and felt a little disorientated. They introduced themselves and told me, 'You're in St Patrick's mental hospital.' My mind instantly cast me back to one of my favourite ever films, *Shutter Island*. This film is based in a mental institution, painting both the institution and the patients within it in a very dark light – people in dark, dreary rooms, strapped into straightjackets, head-butting the walls. I had always believed that this was the reality of a mental hospital.

This thought woke me right up, and I sat upright in bed, eyes wide and fear coursing through my body. 'It's okay, Shane. We're here to help you,' one of the nurses said. I still hadn't said anything at this point, but the thoughts kept coming, bizarre ones at that – including a fear that they were going to put me in a straightjacket and lock me into a padded cell. To this day, I still smile when I think of how little I knew then about mental health services, and mental health in general for that matter.

As if my thoughts weren't already in overdrive, one of the nurses said, 'We're just going to take your bloods, Shane,' as she produced a syringe from her pocket. I gave her permission, but reluctantly. Blood sample taken, the nurses invited me to go to the breakfast area, where the rest of the patients from the Dean Swift Ward were. My guard immediately went up, and I politely declined, requesting that I had my breakfast in my room. I had a preconception of what the other patients would be like, and felt that I wouldn't belong. I wasn't 'crazy'.

It was a real shame that I had such a negative idea of what these patients would be like, because after some back-and-forth between myself and the nurses, I made my way down the corridor toward the breakfast room and was in for a reality check. As I entered the room, I was the object of attention of all the patients. There were whispers of 'he's new' as I made my way to my seat. I was terrified as I sat down, unable to make eye contact with anyone around me.

I was sitting, looking down between my legs when a hand appeared right in front of my eyeline. I peered up to see a smiling patient offering her hand in welcome to the hospital. 'The first few days are always the toughest. It gets better though,' she said. This gesture of kindness eased m nerves somewhat, allowing me to pick my head up from between my legs and gaze across the room, where twelve other patients were sitting.

I scanned around the room, and almost every other patient made eye contact with me, nodding and wearing a welcoming smile. I was a nineteen-year-old boy in a place I'd never been before, with little choice in the matter, and these welcoming, friendly faces helped to calm me. I was naturally still apprehensive in making conversation as breakfast was placed in front of me. As quickly as the bowl of porridge was placed down, I had it eaten and was on my way back to my room.

I had a few moments to myself before the nurse on duty came into my room. I began to ruminate, and fairly soon panic began to set in. 'I need to get out of here, I need to get out of here,' I said. It was an indication of how little control I had over my emotions – a few minutes earlier, sitting at the breakfast table, I had felt fairly content with my surroundings.

A nurse came in to check up on me, only to find me in a flood of tears. She consoled me for a few moments. When the tears began to run dry, she let me know my parents were on their way to see me, and that I'd be meeting the doctor that would be assigned to me for the duration of my stay. She continued, 'it might be better for you to come out to the communal area and get to know some of the patients.' I promptly declined the offer.

The nurse sat by my bedside until it was time to meet my doctor. She brought me to the top of the corridor, through the communal area and into the meeting room where the doctor was. I didn't know what to expect. Around this time, I found it hard to attach any emotions to things, but making my way to the meeting, I certainly could. My heart felt like it was about to come out of my chest, my palms were sweating and I was constantly scanning around me, finding it hard to fix my gaze on anything.

Now I was greeted by a very well-dressed, unintimidating figure, with a voice that would put even the most nervous of patients at ease. I find it difficult to recall much of our conversation, but one detail jumped out at me. This was to do with the average length of time patients generally spend in St Pat's. Other things he was saying were breezing over my head, but when he mentioned this topic, my attention was right with him. It was as though he was talking in slow motion as he uttered the words 'two to four weeks'. Two to four weeks! I was in shock. I refused to accept it. 'I won't be staying for that long. I have an All Ireland semi-final in three days' time,' I said bluntly.

'Shane, you've gone through a traumatic time over the last while. You need to deal with this first,' he said.

I sat there stubbornly, arms folded, shaking my head at anything else he had to say. I still had tunnel vision at this point, believing football was really the only important thing in my life. I simply couldn't see that my life had come to the point where it was a matter of life or death if I didn't face up to the inner turmoil I was experiencing.

I left the meeting filled with anger. My parents were sitting in the communal area, but I walked straight passed them and back to my room. They went in and spoke to the doctor as a nurse came to my bedside again. Soon, my anger switched to despair and the tears began to flow once more. All I wanted was for my problems to disappear and to return to a normal life.

My parents finished the meeting with my doctor and they joined me in my room. The nurse left us to give us privacy. As soon as the nurse shut the door behind her, I said, 'I'm playing that match, Dad'. I couldn't accept where I was and the sheer amount of work I had ahead of me to iron out the two years of inner trauma. 'Dessie will be coming in tomorrow and you can talk to him about it then. Until then, try to forget about it and relax,' my dad said. My mam placed my gear bag on the bed, saying, 'Do you want me to help you unpack and put these away into your wardrobe?' 'No. I won't be here for long,' I said forcefully.

I'm sure it was difficult for my parents to look at their nineteen-year-old son, desperately needing help but refusing to accept that fact. My mam didn't try to argue with me. We took a trip out to the small garden that was visible from the window of my bedroom, staying out there until it was time for them to go, as the patients were called in for lunch. They said their goodbyes and told me they would be back in the morning, after breakfast with Dessie.

Once again, I didn't stay long in the dining area. As therapies weren't going to begin for another few days, to allow for a 'settling-in period', there was potential for me to be left sitting with all the negative thoughts that were swirling around in my head. However, the nurses obviously knew how to deal with new patients, and were aware of the amount of free time patients are given in their first few days. They made sure not to allow me too much time alone, knowing that I'd spend it ruminating. They acted as not only a distraction, but also a means of communication with any questions I had about the hospital – believe me, there were many, due to my distorted perception of a mental hospital. A particular concern of mine was what the hospital was like during the night. A nurse I talked to gave me an overview of what my first night would look like. 'Lights out' would be at 10pm, when most patients would go to their rooms and settle in for the night. Patients could stay out in the communal area, where there were chairs and bean bags, if they wished, to sit and watch television. There would be nurses on night duty, doing hourly check-ups on each room. I could call any one of them if I needed to talk during the night. This information put me much more at ease.

That night, as I settled into bed, I found it difficult to erase the harrowing images I had imagined prior to this. The beginning of the night went exactly as described. I sat upright in my bed with my headphones on, listening to the playlist that had served me so well prior to my admission to the hospital. Then, just after midnight as I recall, I heard what sounded like a blood-curdling scream, coming from a room not too far from mine. I lowered the volume on my headphones. There was silence. Then, after a few moments of silence, another scream. It sounded as though someone was being beaten. I sat still, paralysed with fear, then I shouted, 'Nurse, nurse!'

My bedroom door opened, the light from the hallway shining in. I asked what the commotion was. There was another scream, which felt like it was closer, though really that was only because my door was now open. 'What's going on?' I asked, as my body began to tremble. The nurse came in and sat at the end of bed, saying, 'One of the patients is having difficulty sleeping. It's okay, one of the nurses is seeing to them now.' 'Tell me what's going on,' I demanded, not entirely believing the explanation I was being given. 'Okay. One of the patients is having a panic attack. It's all being taken care of.' 'Can you lock my door?' I asked, worried that someone might come into my room. 'We can't,' she replied. There were, in fact, no locks on the doors, for the safety of the patients. 'You're in safe hands, Shane. We're only down the corridor. Try to get some sleep,' she said. She left the room, leaving the door slightly ajar. The screams had stopped, but I didn't get much sleep that night, and my gaze hardly left the door.

The following morning after breakfast, while I was sitting in my room, my parents and Dessie arrived. They asked how my first night had gone. I was still in a state of shock and felt that I couldn't open up to them about how it really was; I simply said, 'It was fine.' All I was thinking about was the All Ireland semi-final, now only two days away. I didn't waste any time bringing the conversation around to the match. 'Have you cleared it with the hospital to let me out to play the game?' I asked Dessie.

My parents and Dessie looked to the ground awkwardly. Then Dessie broke the news that I wasn't prepared for. 'I've spoken to your parents, team management and doctors. We think it's best you don't play this weekend, Shane,' he said. I scrambled to register what had just been said. 'But why?' I asked. My parents and Dessie talked about all I had been through, but how could I understand what they were saying? Football was all that I knew.

It was all I identified with. To be told that I couldn't do what I loved and what was pretty much my only source of happiness over the last two years was hard to come to terms with. I wasn't angry; I wasn't sad. I was merely numb, confused. We sat a while longer. However, I was unresponsive for the rest of their stay.

I returned to the Dean Swift Ward, where the reality of my situation was becoming clearer as the day went on. I hadn't undergone any therapies yet, as I was still in the 'settling-in' period. This meant I hadn't got the tools or resources yet to deal with it all. I didn't feel like opening up when the nurses came to my side. They offered a listening ear, but I didn't feel like airing my thoughts.

Night time approached, and my mind went into overdrive. The nurses came by my room every hour to do their check-ups. At one point, the nurse on duty was greeted by me in my room at the edge of my bed. My mind was fixated on the thought that the only thing that had given me happiness over the last few years had been taken away from me. The suicidal ideations I'd had in recent months were bubbling away in my mind again. I thought, 'If I can't play football, what reason have I to live?'

I continued to weep as the nurse attended to me. She tried to put it into perspective for me, explaining that I was there to face issues that were going on in my head so that I could begin to enjoy life again. However, I simply couldn't see her point of view, such was the cloudiness in my head. We sat for hours, with the nurse doing most of the talking, as I sat with my head bowed, tears streaming from me. I was exhausted by the time the tears began to dry. I got back into bed, tucking myself in beneath the covers. My body was heavy, energy gone; I had nothing left in me. I knew I would have to face up to it all again the following day, but I didn't know how much I had left to give.

The following morning, my mood hadn't improved. I struggled through the day, desperately searching for the slightest bit of happiness to enter my body. My parents and Stephanie came to visit in the afternoon. However, this didn't lift my mood. I sat there in deep thought on the bed, as they engaged in conversation around me. I searched for a hint of light, any brief respite from the pain I was in, but none materialised. My thoughts were dark and distorted, and my hope was dwindling. I failed to recognise that the light in my life was sitting right next to me that afternoon.

As my parents and Stephanie's stay came to an end, my dad said he would be back the following afternoon with my two best friends, Karl and Moe, to watch the semi-final. The light that I was searching for had now appeared in front of me. As tough as it was facing up to not playing in the game the following day, I was now placing all my hope on my teammates getting over the line, so that I could return for the All Ireland final two weeks later. This was more distorted, irrational thinking. Over the past two years, I had failed to get a grip on my ever-worsening depression, to the point that I now found myself engaging in suicidal ideations. I was three days into my stay in St Patrick's mental hospital, and yet to begin any therapy, suicidal ideations never too far away and yet, despite all this, I still thought I should concentrate on football.

I woke up in good spirits the next day – Saturday, 19 April, All Ireland semi-final day – which was very much welcomed. My lift in mood even saw me engage in conversation at the breakfast table with some other patients. I eagerly awaited the arrival of Karl, Moe and my dad. I set my laptop up on the bedside table with the link to the game ready and waiting, so as not to miss a second of the action.

Karl, Moe and my dad arrived at my bedroom door. It was Karl and Moe's first time to visit me since my admission four days prior, and I could see the worry on their faces as they slowly made their way into the room. They stood awkwardly at the edge of my bed before I offered them a seat on the bed next to me. 'Don't be shy, lads,' I said. My dad took what became his customary seat on the red leather chair in the corner of the room. I'm sure the two lads had burning questions to get off the tips of their tongues, but they would have to wait, as the game was about to begin.

It was a cagey affair, with Cavan leading by two points going into the break. During half time, my Dad paced up and down the corridor. He's naturally nervous when it comes to matches, but the added prospect of me potentially returning for the final should Dublin get over the line had him like this. Ironically, me being the patient, I was the calmest, offering Karl and Moe a cup of tea from the trolley in the communal area. 'So, how has it been?' Moe awkwardly said as I came in with the tea. Naturally, my two best friends were worried for me and I was aware of this. I felt that I didn't want to burden them with too many details of my first four days, so I gave them a fairly generic answer. 'It's been okay, I know it'll be tough, but I'll get through.' They probably believed me, especially as they had caught me in a good mood on this day.

Soon the match was back underway, and my dad was back from his nervous walk of the corridors. The second half didn't begin as planned, and Cavan opened up a four-point lead. My mind wandered during this period, as a cloud of guilt came over me. 'I've let down my teammates,' I said internally, as the game seemed like it could slip away from us. However, a strong third quarter saw us close the deficit to the narrowest of margins. Cavan responded with a point, but a trio of scores late on meant our place in the final was confirmed, as we came out 0-11 to 0-10 victors! My dad and I embraced after the final whistle, and at that moment I cemented in my mind a determination to return for the final two weeks later, completely ignoring the fact that I hadn't even begun to dig into the heart of my problems over the last two years.

Delving into the root of my troubles began the following Monday, 21 April. I had mixed feelings about starting therapy. One part of me was excited to begin, as I wanted a quick fix to the problems I had ignored for so long. Little did I know, however, how much work was ahead of me. Looking back, I hadn't thought of my situation logically at all – I expected that in a matter of one or two sessions, the psychologist could rid me of two years of the most harrowing thoughts you could imagine.

In another part of my mind, I still couldn't erase the preconceptions I had of mental hospitals. The disturbing notions that were swirling around in my head were amusing in retrospect: I pictured a cold, dark, wet room, with a worn chair some distance from where the psychologist would be. The psychologist I pictured had spiky grey hair, was wearing a lab coat and looked pretty unstable himself. The patient was receiving electric shock therapy, and the psychologist laughed as each bolt of current ran through the patient's body.

These were the thoughts that engulfed my mind on this Monday afternoon as I was guided out of the Dean Swift Ward by a nurse. We walked down a long corridor as these images flashed in front of me. As the nurse knocked on the door, it became a projector screen for the movie in my head. The silver door handle seemed to be turning in slow motion.

The door swung open and, to my surprise and relief, the scene I had envisioned couldn't have been further from reality. This psychologist, much like the doctor before, had a soft, comforting tone to her voice. This was the first thing I noted as she showed me to a seat, which wasn't worn or a great distance from where she would sit. Taking a deep breath, I took in my surroundings, which were warm and welcoming, a far cry from what I had imagined. The psychologist had a relaxed demeanour and she smiled broadly. We sat down, and spoke generally to begin with. I began to recount all that I had gone through in the previous two years.

One moment particularly stands out in my memory from this session, and this was the moment when I was officially diagnosed. Towards the end of the one-hour session, having spoken about various incidents, the psychologist told me that she was assured of her diagnosis – I had 'depression'. The immediate feeling was one of relief. I had finally been told what 'it' was. Even though I really had no idea what 'depression' actually meant, it was good to know that I could finally place a label on 'it'.

I returned to the Dean Swift Ward with a strange feeling. Although this wasn't the first time I had spoken up about my difficulties, having verbalised some of them to my parents and Dessie among others, it was the first time I had gone in depth, and attempted to unearth the root causes of my troubles. I found the experience very draining. I felt as though I had come off the pitch after the most gruelling of seventy-minute games. I hadn't been up very long, but I felt like I needed a nap.

I mentioned to the nurses how I felt, and they said it was completely normal to feel this way. They said it was a good idea to take a nap. As soon as my head hit the pillow, I was out for the count.

A few hours later, I was woken by a nurse. I felt I could have slept longer, but she told me that my parents and Dessie and Mick were out in the communal area, waiting for me. I quickly got dressed and went out to meet them.

As I had company, I was allowed to go out to the larger canteen area just outside the Dean Swift Ward. I was glad of this, because very quickly I felt like I was becoming institutionalised, being confined to the one small area. I had to remember though that such restrictions were for my own safety.

We sat around a table in the canteen, and soon a conversation about the upcoming final ensued. Dessie and Mick spoke hypothetically about me not playing the game, as though pre-preparing me for a situation I had never even considered. I was still blinded at this point, failing to truly recognise what my life had come to, sitting in a mental hospital, having regular suicidal ideations. All I had seen since the final whistle blew against Cavan two days before was me pulling on the Dublin jersey to play in the All Ireland final. I simply couldn't see their point of view and, quite honestly, was angered that they were talking this way.

I went back to the ward, wishing I hadn't sat down to hear what they had to say. My parents followed into my room, trying to continue the conversation, but I cut them off almost straight away. My dad sat on the chair in the corner of my room and my mam sat at the end of the bed. I sat on the bed, arms folded, staring down between my legs and not making eye contact with either of them. The room was silent. I marinated in anger for some time before that anger switched to despair. Images of the past two years whizzed by in my head, as I told myself, 'If only that didn't happen, I wouldn't be here.'

I began to weep, unable to control the emotions that seemed to be flashing through my head. My parents stayed with me, occasionally offering a warming hand on my back to let me know they were still there. 'It's okay, Shane. Let it all out,' my mam said. I continued to cry until I couldn't anymore.

It was approaching lunch time; usually visitors would only be allowed to stay for the allocated times set out by the hospital. On this day though, the nurses could see that I needed my family more than anything. I joined the other patients in the dining area for lunch, eating it in record time before rejoining my parents in my room. My dad suggested we watch a film on my laptop to take my mind off things, so we did. As far as I can recall, we watched *Coach Carter* on Netflix – one of my favourite films. In recent times, I have realised that it was these simple things that meant the most to me – my sister bringing me for a walk along the cliffs of Howth, the offer of a hand by one of the patients on my first morning in St Patrick's. My parents sitting with me watching a film on Netflix was added to that list. I would compare the feeling I had that day to sitting around the table at Christmas time with the people who meant most to you in your life – that warm, fuzzy feeling deep in your stomach, that's what I felt on this day. The film ended and my parents were on their way shortly after. That day had had the potential to be one of my most difficult to date. However, the nurses allowing my parents to stay with me changed the shape of it all. I slept easy that night.

The following day, I was due to meet my doctor. I didn't wake up in the best of form. I found it hard to deal with my fluctuations in mood. I didn't want to accept that in its essence, this is exactly what depression is – fluctuating mood states. I thought that if my mood took an upturn, then it should continue in that way. 'I should be happy. I should. I should. I should,' became a common theme. This idea was detrimental to my overall mental condition. Instead of accepting that I had simply woken up feeling low, I felt low about feeling low – almost adding insult to injury. This meant that I wasn't best prepared for the news my doctor was about to deliver to me.

It was just before lunch when I met him. A discussion ensued about the care plan being set up for me, all going well, over the next couple of weeks. This included continuing with the work with my psychologist, transitioning into the open ward, taking part in the Young Adult Programme (YAP) and beginning medication to aid me in all of this. This last item set alarm bells off in my head. 'Medication? What do you mean, medication?' All of my senses were now wide awake, eyes widening in fear. 'It's a normal procedure, Shane, prescribing medication for patients who have been diagnosed with depression,' my doctor said in a calming voice. I wasn't calm though. He went on, 'We're prescribing you an antidepressant called Prozac. Seretonin, which is involved in mood regulation, is low in your brain, and Prozac will help to get it back to a normal level.'

'I'm not taking any medication,' I said bluntly. I was never one for taking medication. In years gone past, if I ever had flu or a headache, my mam would immediately disappear off to her medicine cabinet, containing an array of remedies, but I always refused. I don't know whether this was a male thing in me, as if accepting medication was accepting defeat. The doctor tried his level best to get me on side, saying the medication was in my own best interest. I was adamant that I wouldn't take it, but the doctor told me that I was due to start taking Prozac the following morning.

I left the meeting agitated, and refused to sit down to lunch afterwards. Instead, I opted to go back to my room. In an attempt to calm down, I picked up my headphones and made my way out to the garden. I paced the small space with some of my favourite songs playing. I knew deep down that the doctor was right – I needed this medication to aid in my recovery. After a while, my agitation turned to sadness. I grew resigned to taking the medication, though in my head this was accepting defeat.

The day wore on, afternoon quickly becoming evening as my mood continued to decline. The darkness of the night coincided with ever-darkening thoughts. Suicidal ideations were linked with that word 'defeat', which wasn't leaving my mind any time soon. Sleep was hard to come by that night, and each passing hour, the nurse on duty saw my bolt-upright figure sitting in bed, staring ahead as though in a trance. The suicidal ideations only stopped when my body eventually gave in to tiredness at about 3am.

When my head rose from the pillow at 8am the following morning, it was as if someone had pressed play again on the suicidal ideations that were swirling in my head the entire previous evening. The nurse on duty came to the door of my room to tell me it was breakfast time, but I didn't feel like moving. It felt as though the suicidal ideations in my head had me paralysed. 'Shane, are you coming for breakfast?' the nurse asked again. There was only silence from me. She came to the side of my bed and leaned over slightly to my eye level. I glanced at her, shaking my head to refuse the offer of breakfast. 'What's going on for you, Shane?' she asked, now sitting on the side of my bed.

The previous evening I had wanted to speak up, to tell the nurses of the harrowing suicidal ideations that were in my head, but I couldn't, I just couldn't. Now though, I came out with it, perhaps only to get the crippling thoughts out of my head. I couldn't articulate it very well, but I said to the nurse, 'I don't want to do this anymore.' I broke down into tears, and the nurse laid a comforting hand on my back. 'What do you mean, you don't want to do this anymore, Shane?' she asked. My pulse rose; I was almost too afraid to say it. 'I, I, I ...' I struggled to get it out in the open. 'It's okay, Shane,' the nurse said calmly. With my heart rate racing and what I wanted to say flashing before me, I came out with it. 'I want to die,' I said, inconsolably breaking into tears. I sat there for what must have been hours. At one point between all the crying, the nurse who was sitting at the side of my bed went to my bedroom door where another nurse had appeared. They spoke for a few moments.

The nurse that had been by my bedside now let the other nurse take a seat beside me. 'Shane, we have to take what our patients say seriously. In light of what you said this morning, we're going to have to transfer you to the Secure Unit,' she said. 'The Secure Unit,' I echoed, as my stomach turned. My preconceptions of a mental hospital went into overdrive again, telling me internally, 'That's where all the crazy people are.'

In fact, if you stood in the communal area of the Dean Swift Ward and looked beyond the reception area, you could see part of the Secure Unit. I remember asking another patient on one of my first days what area of the hospital that was, and his expression said it all. 'That's the Secure Unit,' he replied, shaking his head as if to suggest, 'You don't want to go in there.' However, this was now my reality.

Everything moved pretty quickly. The nurses told me to pack up my stuff, which didn't take long as I hadn't unpacked in the first place, and we made our way across to the Secure Unit. The layout was much like that of the Dean Swift Ward – a long corridor with rooms on either side, a communal area, a garden and an open ward almost like a fish bowl with four or five beds in it, curtains segregating each 'room'. I was brought to a vacant bed in the open ward to get everything 'checked off'. The nurses from the Dean Swift Ward placed my belongings by my bedside. The nurses on duty in the Secure Unit took it from there.

I was informed that during my stay here, my laptop and phone would be in their possession. This was to eliminate any distractions and the risk of social media for example having a negative influence on me. I didn't mind this too much – I had deleted all social media from my phone in the first few days and the laptop was only used to watch Netflix, something I could live without.

They then requested that all laces or strings be removed from my footwear and clothing. I looked at the nurse as if she was joking. How could it be a joke though? Only hours before, I had said that I wanted to die. This was a necessary measure to protect me. I removed the laces from my four pairs of runners, and the strings from any item of clothing that had them. Now I was brought down to my room, at the end of the corridor on the left. The room was similar to the one I had had in the Dean Swift Ward.

Only a few moments later, I was called into the dining area for lunch. The prejudice I had felt walking into the dining area of the Dean Swift Ward on my first morning was back again as I made my way up the corridor to sit down for lunch in the Secure Unit. I timidly made my way over to two seats that were available on the very far side of the room. The vacant seat beside me was taken up by a thin, fair-haired young man. He introduced himself and asked, 'What are you in for?' It was a question I wasn't expecting, and he asked it as if he were asking the time. I hesitantly answered, 'Depression, what about you?' 'Bipolar,' he said casually. I didn't know how to respond, and simply nodded my head in acknowledgement.

Lunch was placed in front of us. One thing was different, however – it was served on plastic plates, with plastic cutlery. I turned to the patient I'd just been talking to. 'Not what you're used to,' he smiled. I nervously smiled back. I hurriedly ate my lunch, feeling uneasy about my surroundings.

Back in my room, I didn't have too much time to think, as my parents and Stephanie arrived not long afterwards. I embraced them one by one as they came in. My dad and Stephanie have always been good at keeping their emotions in check, but my mam's facial expression said it all.

I wanted to speak about something else away from football and the hospital, simply to switch off. My Dad isn't shy of telling a story or two, about his childhood or soccer trips away with his old club, Glasnevin FC. As a family, we're usually quick to cut his stories short, as they notoriously go on for a long time, veering off on tangents, but on this day this wasn't the case. I sat intently listening to every word my dad had to say, engrossed in the stories he had to tell. My mam and Stephanie occasionally cut in and had their say, but I probably said no more than five words in what must have been two hours of storytelling. I was content, having so recently been so low and lost. In your darkest times, it's very often the most simple of things that bring you the most joy – this was the case on this day, as I sat with the people who meant the most to me in my life.

A couple of days passed. While sleep was hard to come by, with the constant noise going on in my head and peculiar sounds heard from down the corridor, there was time for some lighter moments during the day. On Friday, 25 April, my parents came to visit. I wasn't allowed out to the garden unless I was accompanied by a nurse or, as on this day, by my parents. My dad had brought along a football so that we could have a kick around like the 'good oul' days'. My mam sat on a bench while my dad and I played with the football. There was another patient in the garden, accompanied by a nurse of course, not far from us. My mam went silent, and I peered over my shoulder to see why. She was gazing over at the other patient, and then she turned to look at me, measuring me up and down. She had a burning question on her mind: 'Shane, the patients are in their own clothing, just like the visitors. How can the nurses distinguish between the two?' 'Oh, that's easy,' I told her. 'All they have to do is look down at our shoes – the patients have no laces!' There was a moment of silence, and then a slightly nervous laugh, as though my parents were unsure whether or not this was appropriate. We have laughed about this moment many times since – it was funny, but it captured the reality of the situation I was in at that time.

The time I spent in the Secure Unit, with nothing around me to occupy my mind, gave me an opportunity to reflect. At times this was both dark and difficult, and I often found it hard to get a handle on the thoughts racing through my head. The nurses helped me out of those spiralling thoughts through the medium of talk therapy.

On Saturday, 26 April, my mind was free, which allowed for probably my biggest breakthrough of all during my time in St Patrick's. This shift began with me sitting at the edge of my bed, staring at my lace-less shoes, thinking about how I had got here. From a very young age, I was given a talent that encompassed many sports, in particular Gaelic football. This placed me up on a pedestal among my peers from very early on in my life, a pedestal I never wanted to be on. This pedestal grew even larger when I went into secondary school, with my continuing successes in sport. When my Dublin football career really started, I was seen as this guy living an idyllic life, representing my county in front of 80,000 people in Croke Park. Meanwhile, I was embarking on a two-year journey into ever-worsening depression. I felt that I couldn't tell anyone about this, as my life was supposed to be perfect.

That was until now. Being admitted to St Patrick's made me realise that I wasn't the only one going through such experiences. There are thousands of people suffering in silence, just like I did, unable to see the wood for the trees.

Instead of hiding away from the pedestal so many people saw me on, why not stand proud on top of it and illuminate the path for others? Let them know that the guy living the 'idyllic' life can also go through difficulty in his life.

This was the journey my mind went on, finishing with two conclusions: firstly, I couldn't play in the upcoming All Ireland final – I had to focus on my recovery in hospital; and secondly, I would make my whereabouts and what I was being treated for public knowledge. My parents visited me that afternoon and I told them the decisions I'd made. The next step was to inform Dessie. I wouldn't have to wait long, as he was due to visit me in a couple of days' time.

The following day, Sunday, I met with my doctor. He was satisfied that I was no longer a danger to myself, which meant I moved back into the Dean Swift Ward that evening. The next afternoon, Dessie came to visit. Naturally, I was nervous about what I was about to tell him. I had spent most of the morning going back and forth in my head about whether it was the right thing to do. After all, I'd spent the previous two years keeping all of this hidden. Now I was about to let the whole world know. But when I thought of the thousands of silent sufferers out there, I realised that with the privileged position I was in, I could make a real impact.

I met Dessie in the main canteen, around the corner from the Dean Swift Ward. My parents were there too. As we sat down, Dessie asked, 'How are you getting on, Shane?' I didn't waste any time in getting to the point. I took one deep breath and came out with it. I hardly made eye contact with him as I spoke, instead fixing my gaze on the table as I concentrated on recounting exactly the journey my mind had gone on in the last couple of days. I finished with one deep exhale, peering up to see his reaction. Smiling broadly, he said, 'I'm delighted to hear that, Shane.'

I didn't know it at the time, but my parents and Dessie knew I wasn't going to be playing any part in the final, just six days away. They hadn't known how to break the news to me, because I was like a frog in a well, looking up. Now they wouldn't have to have that difficult conversation with me.

We decided that Dessie would make a statement at the All Ireland final press preview in two days' time, detailing where I was and what I was being treated for. We spoke about the potential reaction that this would provoke. Dessie advised me to stay off any social media, which wasn't an issue, as I'd already cut myself off from the outside world. As Dessie left, his parting message was, 'You're doing a great thing here, Shane.'

I returned to the ward, feeling like the weight of the world had come off my shoulders. Things were slowly beginning to take shape now, and some sparks of light were coming back into my darkened mind. I had realised that maybe there was a life outside football!

The following Tuesday, 29 April, I had a meeting with my doctor. He filled me in on his plans for me over the next while, and how he thought I was progressing. He asked if there was anything I'd like in addition to what they were already offering. My answer was quick and simple: 'Yes, an open field.' I hadn't been able to do any exercise here, apart from the occasional walk in the very small garden. This wasn't enough for me. If there was one thing I had learned over the previous two years, it was that physical exercise made me feel like I was worth a little something. The doctor replied that they would discuss the possibility of 'accompanied leave' – they would let me know by the end of the day. For the rest of the day, the only thing on my mind was the possibility of 'accompanied leave'.

After dinner, I was out in the garden, nervously pacing around with my headphones on. A nurse appeared at the door to the garden, gesturing for me to come over. As I removed my headphones and walked over, I noticed that she began to smile, grinning from ear to ear. 'I've got good news, Shane,' she said. 'You've been granted accompanied leave.' I was overjoyed, and didn't waste any time in letting my parents know, pulling my phone from my pocket to contact them – naturally they were delighted for me. That night, as the nurse on duty was doing her routine room check-ups, she asked, 'What are you planning to do?' 'Find an open field and go for a run,' I said. I knew by her facial expression that this wasn't the answer she was expecting. I guess other patients would go to their favourite restaurant, or go shopping or for coffee with friends. But for me, one thing above all brought me joy – the simple pleasure of physical exercise.

The very next day, Wednesday, 30 April, I was to be let out on accompanied leave. The problems I'd been facing seemed to subside entirely for the day, leading up to getting out. Dessie was to make his public announcement as to my whereabouts that evening, but that didn't concern me at all. Stephanie came to the hospital after dinner time, around 7pm. I had been ready for some time, and sat shamelessly at the edge of my bed, head to toe in my Dublin gear. Before the door had fully swung open, I was standing, gear bag in hand, smiling from ear to ear. I was already making a beeline for the exit door before she could say, 'Are you ready?'

We went out to the car and I put my gear bag into the boot before getting into the front seat. Before she pulled off, I asked Stephanie to wait. I put my hood up, pulling on the strings to reduce my peripheral vision, but still enough to see straight ahead, and cranked the seat back to the fully reclined position. I simply didn't want to see anyone I knew, and didn't want to be seen either. Stephanie pulled off and we were on our way. She suggested we go to the Phoenix Park, and I agreed. Due to my reduced vision, Stephanie updated me on our whereabouts every few moments, probably noticing how uneasy I was along the way.

Soon, we arrived at the car park. I rose from my reclined position, loosened the strings on my hood and peered around. We were at the cricket grounds in the Phoenix Park, which had three Gaelic pitches right next to them, where I had played a few matches before.

I got my football boots from my gear bag in the boot and swiftly put them on. 'Do you want me to come with you, Shane?' Stephanie asked. 'No, it's okay,' I replied, placing my headphones on my head and my hood over them. I made my way up to the top pitch and placed my water bottle to the right hand side of the goal. My sister later recalled that she was hugely nervous watching on from the car – five yards beyond the goal, there were trees and shrubs that made it difficult to see anything beyond that point. She feared I would head that way and disappear, 'making an escape'.

Beginning my warm up, I couldn't have been happier. This was everything I wanted – me, my music and an open field. Of course, here in the Phoenix Park I might have to contend with the occasional deer encroaching on me! I planned to do four 1km time trials, a test that many Gaelic players are familiar with, particularly in the depths of winter. I had downloaded the 'MapMyRun' app, which would keep track of my time and distance. The competitive streak that was ingrained in me meant that I wanted to improve my time for each run.

The end line was my starting point for the run. I measured out 100m from that point and scuffed a mark in the ground with my boot to indicate where to turn back. That mark became my engraving on the famous Phoenix Park grounds for the rest of the time I would spend in hospital.

I began my run. The feeling I experienced for the next forty-five minutes was something I had missed over the last few weeks in hospital. All of my concerns washed away with each long stride I took. I didn't want to be anywhere else in the world in that moment. I was slightly saddened as I finished the last of my four 1km time trials, knowing I'd have to wait for the next day to do it again. However, as I returned to the car with a spring in my step, the overriding feeling was one of euphoria.

As I sat back into the car, Stephanie told me that the Dublin County Board had just released a statement on their website. She turned her phone in my direction to show me the headline: 'Carthy receiving treatment for depression'. I put my hand out to indicate that I'd seen enough. It wasn't that I was ashamed to read the statement – quite the opposite in fact. However, it was enough for me to see the headline to feel a huge weight being lifted off my shoulders. I hoped that my decision to speak out about my personal difficulties could help others in my situation. This thought brought a smile to my face as we made our way back to the hospital.

As my treatment continued, I was still getting used the tiredness I experienced after each session with the psychologist. I understood the reason for this though – I was unravelling thoughts and feelings I had suppressed for two years, bringing them to the surface and dealing with them head on. I confided more in the nurses as the All Ireland final approached, naturally finding difficulty sometimes in dealing with the fact that I wasn't going to be playing.

All Ireland final day, Saturday, 3 May, arrived. It was inevitable that this day would be one of my toughest. My psychologist had suggested that I plan out my day – to have things planned to keep my mind occupied before and after the game. The first thing on my list was to take a trip to the

Phoenix Park in the morning. My mind desperately wanted to pull me into ruminating about the game, which would have led me into a downward spiral. The run gave me a brief respite from the noise in my head.

My dad and I returned to the hospital, where the nurses had very kindly reserved a room for us to watch the game. It was suggested earlier in the week that maybe I shouldn't watch the game, but I very quickly dismissed that notion. There was no way I was going to miss this match. My dad served as a great distraction as we waited for the game to start, filling any silences that might have let me converse negatively in my head. As he did back in the Secure Unit, he filled the air with great stories of his childhood and his days with Glasnevin FC – stories that I'd never heard before.

Then the match was about to begin, and we fixed our gazes on the television. 'Amhrán na bhFiann' played out, and the camera scanned across all of my teammates, standing shoulder to shoulder. I couldn't help but wish I was there for that special moment.

The match got underway. It turned out a very one-sided affair, with Dublin leading 0-14 to 0-01 at half time. I jumped up from my seat at half time and went back to my room to get my headphones. Although I had only had a few sessions with my psychologist, one thing she had got me to work on was recognising when my thoughts were wandering. At these times, I should remove myself from the situation and busy myself with something else, so that I don't begin a spiral of negative emotions.

This is exactly what I was doing here. I stuck on my headphones and paced the garden, listening intently to every word in the music, desperately trying to ignore the dark thoughts that were threatening. It worked quite well, and I regained a steady thought process, ready to rejoin my dad for the start of the second half.

Despite an attempted late revival, with Roscommon raising three green flags in the second half, the game had been over since half time, and Dublin came out nine-point victors. Throughout the game, I had managed to stay relatively calm, keeping a lid on the dark thoughts that were trying their best to engross my mind. However, when the final whistle blew and I saw the joy on all my teammates' faces, that was a moment that I found it difficult. I watched on as the celebrations erupted, and tears started to stream down my face. I bowed my head, focusing my gaze on my legs. I thought to myself, 'There's nothing wrong with me; I could have been there.' This was partly true. Yes, physically I could have been there, but mentally I couldn't have been further from ready.

The negative spiral began, and it got dark quickly. I headed out to the garden again with my headphones, but by this stage, my mind had gone far from any rational thought. The noises got louder and louder as I hunkered down, breaking down in an uncontrollable flow of tears. My dad came over and offered a hand on my back. My mind was dark and clouded as I rose up, embracing my dad for several minutes.

The nurse and my dad helped me back in from the garden, and I staggered to my room. I sat on the edge of my bed until I could cry no more and gradually regained my composure. Hanging over me was the wish that I'd been there, but I also said internally, 'I'm glad that's over.' It was a huge hurdle to overcome and one I found difficult to deal with clearly. However, as day wore into night, my mind began to settle. I knew I'd have to deal with it again in the proceeding days, but I felt I was over the worst of that particular situation.

The week starting Monday, 5 May, saw me continue work with my psychologist, and trips to the Phoenix Park were now a daily occurrence. Now,

I'm an avid coffee drinker, sometimes consuming five to six cups a day – it's fair to say, I like my coffee. There was coffee available within the hospital, but it just didn't compare to my favourites like Costa, Butlers and of course, Starbucks. I was approaching my third week in hospital, and I felt I was becoming so institutionalised that I'd forgotten what a really good coffee tasted like. One evening, after my run in the park, I asked my sister if we could go and get a coffee from one of my three favourite coffee shops. 'No problem,' she replied. She chose Starbucks on College Green in the city centre. I hadn't quite built up the courage yet to face a crowded café, so Stephanie went in and ordered a take away coffee. She returned and I sat up in the car, loosened my hood and took my first sip of the most simple of all coffees, an Americano!

You're probably thinking, what's the significance of this? It's just a cup of coffee. Yes, that's all it is. However, only when you've experienced real inner turmoil do you realise that the most simple of things can mean everything. This little experience – sitting in the car, coffee in hand and my sister by my side – reminded me that my life was worth something.

Although it took a huge amount of mental resolve, my mind remained calm for the entirety of the week. I used the few tools and resources given to me by my psychologist to keep myself in this steady headspace. It seemed that progress was being made. My doctor decided that I could make the move to the Open Unit for the week starting Monday, 12 May.

Monday came and I was ready to transition to the Open Unit. I was brought up to the second floor of the hospital by one of the nurses, to the Kilroot Ward. Naturally, I was nervous, not quite knowing what was behind the two brown doors leading into the new ward. The nurse kindly held open the door as I gingerly made my way through. I was passed over to the nurse on duty in this section of the hospital.

The layout here was different to downstairs. There were no individual rooms; instead, there were six or seven beds in each of the three sections, with curtains segregating each area. Past these sections and the toilet and shower areas was the medication room, where patients came to collect their prescriptions at set times of the day. There was a small communal area with some chairs and a television, and another room with chairs and a television if you didn't wish to sit out in the communal area. Completing the ward was the dining area, visible from outside the room through windows that ran the whole way along.

My 'room' consisted of a bed, a bedside locker and a wardrobe. I wasn't quite comfortable with the fact that all that separated me from the patient next to me was a curtain, as part of me still hung on to the prejudice I had towards other patients. It was a hurdle I would have to overcome, as I had little choice in the matter.

The Open Unit gave patients more responsibility and more freedom. We were allowed to roam any section of the hospital we wished, including access to the larger canteen area and the large garden at the back of the hospital. Check-ups were no longer on an hourly basis; instead, there was one in the morning and one at 10pm. The nurse told me that I would be taking part in the Young Adult Programme (YAP), something my doctor would give me more information on when I met him in a few days' time. There was a lot to take in, and I felt somewhat overwhelmed by it all.

As I settled into my new surroundings, I noted that the majority of the patients were male and of a similar age to me. This was intentional, so that patients would feel comfortable conversing with each other. During the day, other patients in my section very kindly introduced themselves, noting that I was new to the ward. I didn't go into detailed conversations with any of them, but the gesture made me feel somewhat more at ease.

My parents visited a while later, and a trip to the Phoenix Park was very much welcomed, to cleanse the cloudiness in my head from the day's events. I arrived back shortly before the 10pm check-up, as I nervously awaited my first night in the Kilroot Ward. I drew my curtain closed, keeping the lamp, directly above my bed on the wall, on for the time being. I sat there, as though expecting something to happen, probably still showing some mental scars from uneasy nights I had experienced downstairs. In reality, the night passed without incident.

I met my doctor on Wednesday, 14 May. After a couple of days in the Open Unit, I was finding it difficult to cope with all the independent, unstructured time I was being afforded. I was glad when he told me I would be starting the YAP in two days' time. He gave me a brief rundown of what would be involved: The YAP is aimed at eighteen-to-twenty-five-year-olds with any mental health diagnosis. It includes discussions and leisure activities, all delivered via group sessions, with the aim of fostering a sense of 'not being the only one'. I was both excited and apprehensive about starting the programme. I hoped it would bring me further along my recovery path, but I hadn't yet engaged much with other patients, so hearing that everything was done in a group setting did create a certain amount of nervousness.

Following my meeting with the doctor, I returned to my room. I wasn't coping very well with the thoughts coming into my mind though, so I spoke to one of the nurses, highlighting my concerns. She acted as the listening ear I needed, as they almost always did. My mam arrived a little later, and if there was one thing I needed at that moment, it was the ever-reliable open field. I was fearful of being alone again, knowing I would spend the time ruminating. I asked my mam if we could spend more time out than we usually did, and she obliged. We took the long route to the Phoenix Park, or so my mam told me – I couldn't confirm this, as I was again in the reclined position, staring up at the ceiling.

I took my time in everything I did when we eventually arrived. As I slowly walked up to the very top pitch, I broke into a smile, knowing that in a matter of minutes the weight I felt on me would be offloaded. I wasn't wrong either, because as I began to run, it felt like every step I took was cleansing my mind more and more.

My run came to an end and my mam later recalled that I looked ten feet tall returning to the car. We continued to take our time, picking up a coffee in Starbucks on College Green on our way back to the hospital. I had managed to fend off the dark clouds that were threatening earlier in the day, but there were only so many runs and coffee trips I could go on. Eventually I would have to face up to the underlying problems.

The following evening, I was given my YAP timetable by one of the two coordinators of the programme. We spoke for a few minutes before he went on his way. The timetable was like one you might get at the start of a school year. The programme would run from 9am to 2pm, Monday to Friday. I was glad to be starting the next day, as I was struggling with so much independent time. The programme would not only give structure to my day, but I hoped it would give me the skills I was so clearly lacking.

I sat in bed that night, thinking through the positives I hoped would come from the programme. Unsurprisingly, I also thought of the negatives that might come from it. My overriding worry was what the other patients would think of me. 'Will they judge me? Will they think I'm weird? Will they think I'm different?'

The next morning, Friday, 16 May, I headed down the stairs towards the front of the hospital, to where my first session was. According to the timetable, it would be a group discussion, due to begin at 9am. I arrived fifteen minutes early to avoid the feared late walk in. The door was locked, although I could peer through the small window – a smallish room, with chairs arranged in a semi-circle.

Footsteps came from up the corridor, and a young man appeared – clearly another patient, judging by his age. He confidently approached me, extending his arm and introducing himself. Other patients appeared down the corridor, in a jovial mood, laughing and joking as they came nearer. They were obviously all familiar with one another, which added to my nerves, as I worried that I wouldn't fit in.

The coordinator arrived a few moments later, and I hastily followed him into the room, choosing a seat in the very corner. The other patients came in and took their seats. The coordinator began: 'Today, we'll be doing CBT, but before we get started on that, I have to introduce the newcomer to the programme.' Although I had no idea what 'CBT' was, my immediate concern was that I might have to speak. 'Do you want to introduce yourself, or will I?' he asked. 'You can,' I said, letting out a huge exhale of relief. The introduction he gave was brief, but he concluded with, 'Shane is also a Dublin footballer.' I knew he meant well, but I would have preferred to steer away from my identity as a sporting figure. I wanted to be recognised as Shane the person before being placed up on a pedestal like so often. I could see as he mentioned 'footballer', I was the immediate centre of attention in the room. Thankfully, he didn't labour the point.

Our Cognitive Behavioural Therapy (CBT) session got underway. During the session, I learned what CBT was – it involves understanding problems in terms of the relationships between feelings, thoughts and behaviours. It focuses on factors that might maintain problems in the 'here and now'. It seeks to identify beliefs from the past that might keep problems going in the present. I was allowed to offer my personal experience on topics that were brought up, but I decided that I'd just observe, it being my first day.

As I sat listening to the conversation going on in the group, I was taken aback by the sheer honesty of those who spoke. I could relate to a number of things that various patients spoke about. This was the start of realising that what I was experiencing was happening in other people's lives too. The session came to a close, and the coordinator told us what our afternoon leisure activity was going to be – pottery. 'How is pottery going to help in my recovery?' I wondered.

After the CBT session, we had an hour until the start of the pottery class. I was pretty sceptical about it, and asked some of the others if they found pottery classes beneficial to their recovery. One patient, in fact, said they found it 'therapeutic' and a simple way to 'switch off'. Others simply said they preferred it to sitting up in the room ruminating – this was something I could relate to! Still not entirely convinced, I made my way down to the pottery room with some of the others. The class got underway and I quickly realised two things: firstly, I wasn't very good at pottery; and secondly, I didn't find it therapeutic. Nevertheless, I found the social aspect of it very worthwhile. It was the first time I had really engaged with any of the patients and it allowed me to regain a sense of reality while also removing the prejudice I still had towards them. I went away from my first day of the YAP with an appreciation of things I had simply never exposed myself to before.

The next few days had the potential to be difficult. It was the weekend, which meant not only were my doctor and psychologist not on site, but the YAP wasn't running either. And difficult is exactly what these days turned out to be. It came to a head on Sunday, as I spent most of the morning leant over on the side of my bed, my head in my hands and tears streaming from my cheeks to the floor beneath me. I had found it hard for much of the previous day to filter the thoughts coming into my head. The thoughts were situations that my psychologist and I had brought to the surface earlier on in the week. Although we'd rooted out potential causes of my troubles, I simply wasn't equipped to deal with long periods on my own. I had managed to keep the tears at bay through Saturday, using physical exercise and talk therapy as an escape, but there was inevitably going to be a time when I was left to my own thoughts. That time came on Sunday. A nurse came to my bedside, but I quickly dismissed her, saying, 'I want time alone.' You would think this was the time when I needed someone by my side. There comes a point, however, when you get fed up of talking, talking and talking, when all you want to do is wallow in your own tears.

A few moments later, out of the corner of my tear-filled eye, I noticed a figure standing over me. I shouted in frustration, 'I told you I want to be alone!' I peered up, expecting to see the nurse that had been at my bedside moments earlier. It wasn't her though. The figure standing over me was, in fact, Mick Galvin. He had kindly taken time out of his day to pay me a visit, not expecting that he would be greeted in this way! He sat down on the chair beside my bed as I retreated, embarrassed, to the hunched-over position I had been in. A voice in my head said, 'He has come here to see you, and you're like this,' adding to my distress.

As much as I wanted the tears to stop and to engage in conversation with Mick, I couldn't. Mick later recalled that he sat there for over an hour without any conversation coming from my side – through no fault of mine, he added. My frustrations grew as the spiral continued. It became abundantly clear to Mick that I wasn't in the headspace to converse, and he asked, 'Will I leave you be, Shane?' I couldn't even pull myself together to answer, but that was an answer in itself.

A nurse came to my bedside as Mick laid a gentle hand on my back, as he said his goodbyes. The nurse asked, 'Is there anything I can do for you, Shane?' 'I just want to sleep,' I muttered. She asked me to come into the nurses' office, metres from where my bed was. I didn't even have the energy to pick my head up, looking down at the floor as I stood and trudged along behind her. She took out my file and informed me that the doctor had pre-scribed me a tablet called Phenergan when needed. The nurse told me that this is a sleeping aid. At this point I didn't care what I was given, so long as it put me to sleep. 'Is it okay if we give you that?' she asked, and I nodded my head in agreement. The nurse gave me a cup of water and the tablet, and told me it would take about forty minutes to get into my system. I took it as she showed me back to my bed, and soon I was asleep.

Almost twelve hours later, I was woken by one of the nurses. I was groggy and disorientated, and took a few minutes to get my bearings before I staggered up to the dining area. I returned to my room a short while later, still feeling the effects of the Phenergan I had taken. I sat listening to music, awaiting the time for YAP, due to begin at 9am. However, a nurse appeared by my bedside, telling me that the doctor wanted to see me at nine. This was curious, as I was only scheduled to meet him on the Wednesday.

Nine o'clock came and I went to see the doctor. I wasn't prepared for what was to come. He asked how my first week had gone in the Open Unit and I answered honestly, outlining some of the difficulties I had faced throughout the week. He suggested that maybe it was best that I return to the Dean Swift Ward, as perhaps I wasn't as ready to cope in the Open Unit as he had thought. I knew he was right, having thought the same at various stages in the week, but it was difficult to accept this fact. I saw it as a failure, and failure was something I didn't deal with very well. The doctor said that I needed to take 'one step back to take two steps forward'. I didn't cope very well with hearing this news, fighting to hold back the tears.

The meeting concluded and I went back to my room to gather my belongings. I tried to pack up as quickly as possible, so that the others weren't aware that I was on the move. I was accompanied from the second floor back down to the Dean Swift Ward, hanging my head in shame and not making eye contact with any of the other patients. I was passed over from one nurse back to the other. Taking note of my demeanour, she quite quickly showed me to my room.

I didn't have the luxury of my own room as I had the last time I was there. Instead, I was shown to a room with five or six beds in it, with curtains to separate them. There was a window that looked out to the car park at the front of the hospital. I wasn't afforded accompanied leave on this day either, as the doctor felt that I needed to settle in again.

The nurses were in more frequent contact now, offering a listening shoulder if I so wished, but I was fed up talking, preferring to be left with my own thoughts. The only time I did decide to speak was when Stephanie came to visit that afternoon, but even at that as she later recalled, 'You were physically in front of me, but mentally you were elsewhere.' We spent some time out in the garden area, playing with the football. Then we sat down to watch a film on Netflix, but my mind simply couldn't concentrate on the here and now. Stephanie left a short while later.

I struggled as day faded into night, still refusing the offer of a listening ear from the nurses. I confined myself to my room, not wanting to engage with any patients, purely out of shame. Sleep was hard to come by that night, with my mind racing. My body gave in before my mind, eventually getting to sleep, but knowing I'd have to face it all again the next day.

Morning came, and I was due to attend the YAP. Patients in the Secure Unit or the Dean Swift Ward don't normally attend the YAP, but the previous day, the doctor had decided it would be in my best interests for me to continue with the YAP. Initially I was glad about this decision, but on this morning, my mind was clouded and I was reluctant to attend the programme. I realised though that if I didn't attend the programme, I'd be left in my room to ruminate.

I went along to the programme, but much like the day before, I was there physically but not mentally. One of the other patients asked, 'Where were you yesterday?' I wanted to make an excuse, but I was so mentally drained that I found it a real struggle. I came out with the truth, and there was no judgement from the other patient as I told him. The only judgement was coming from my own mind. I sat in with the group discussion, but I can't recall to this day what was brought up, as my mind seemed to drift further and further from my body.

I do recall, however, returning to the Dean Swift Ward after the morning's session. There was an hour to spare before the afternoon session, but I had no intention of going. As I sat up on my bed, suicidal ideations began to enter my ever-darkening mind. I got up to draw my curtains, something patients weren't allowed to do during the daytime. I sat back up on my bed, removing my shoes and placing them beside me on the bed.

From this point, my mental and physical actions were independent. I was merely a spectator to my physical actions. I removed the laces from my shoes, tying them together to make a longer string to fit around the curtain rail. All the while, my mind was screaming, 'Stop, stop, stop!' I was powerless though. Images of my family flashed through my head. This was the first time this had happened – every other time I'd been at this point, I had failed to register a thought about my family.

Before I could go any further, the sound of the curtains being drawn open startled me. The nurse quickly stripped the laces from my lap, forcefully asking, 'What are you doing, Shane?' I didn't answer. It was another few moments before I was coherent enough to realise what I was doing, while the nurse stood over me awaiting an answer. I stared ahead of me, looking at my laces in the nurse's hand. I broke down at this point, and it wasn't long before anger coursed through my body. Another uncontrollable action took hold of me, as I punched the white metal grate covering the window a number of times, before being held back by the nurse.

I retreated to my bed, sobbing. I pleaded with the nurse, 'It wasn't my intention to do what it looks like,' as I knew the likelihood was that I would be put back into the Secure Unit following this. The truth was that it hadn't been my intention to die by suicide, but that was going to be very hard to explain with what the nurse had seen when she drew the curtains back. The tears soon ran dry, and I tried to explain myself to the nurse. I kept pleading that they shouldn't put me into the Secure Unit; that I wasn't a danger to myself.

She replied that she trusted me. I wasn't going to be placed in the Secure Unit, but my curtains were to be kept open at all times, and a very close eye was going to be on me from that point. She added that the situation was going to be flagged with my doctor for the next time I was due to meet him, and what he decided to do following that was out of her control.

The nurse advised me to have a lie down, to 'relax my mind'. We could speak further later on in the evening if needed. I lay down on the bed, mentally exhausted from what had occurred. I peered down at my scuffed and bloodied knuckles, thankful for the intervention made by the nurse.

The next day, I was nervous about the potential outcome of the meeting I was due to have with my doctor. My nerves were eased moments after entering the meeting room, as the doctor got straight to the point. 'We won't be moving you into the Secure Unit. Although, so that we can keep a closer eye on you, accompanied leave has been suspended for the rest of this week,' he said. I was grateful, and relieved.

A little later that day, I had a session with the psychologist. We spoke about the event that had occurred. One thing we talked about was the fact that I had reached a point where talking about my emotions wasn't an issue anymore. In fact, I was experiencing times when I had thoughts or feelings to get off my chest, but was fed up of talking, so I kept it within. My mind was like a volcano – every time I kept a thought inside, the pressure would build. Eventually, the pressure got too much and the volcano erupted. The event from the previous day was an example of this.

The psychologist said that it was completely normal not to want to talk about my feelings all the time. However, keeping them within was not advisable. Instead of doing this, she made a simple suggestion: I should write the thoughts down. I came away from the session keen to put this into practice. I returned to the YAP the following day and began to make some real headway into my overall recovery.

I received a very special phone call on Saturday, 24 May. It was after lunchtime, and I had just returned to the hospital, having spent the afternoon in the Phoenix Park with Stephanie. I was putting away some clothes Stephanie had brought up for me when my phone rang on the bedside locker. It was my other sister, Mairead. She was ringing me all the way from New York, where she had spent the past few days with her boyfriend, Colin. She asked how I was getting on. I returned the question, and she said that she had 'exciting news'. She left a long, drawn-out pause, then, 'Colin and I are engaged!' she said in an excited, high-pitched voice. She filled me in on all the details, as I listened to how thrilled she sounded on the other end of the phone. She went on to tell me that I was the first person they had let know.

This phone call was a real glint of light in an otherwise dark and bleak time. It gave me more reason to believe that life was worth living; that maybe there was a brighter and better future ahead, a future that the cloudiness in my head wouldn't yet allow me to see.

The following week saw me add to what I called my 'mental health toolbox'. The YAP allowed me, through the medium of conversation, to learn what worked for other individuals and take from that. The group sessions opened up conversations I'd never been exposed to before. As my mind continued to clear, my engagement in these sessions increased, and I took more away from them as a result.

My progress had been noted by the nurses, my psychologist and my doctor. So much so that on Wednesday, 28 May, nine days after making the, to my mind shameful, walk down to the Dean Swift Ward, I was now on my way back up to the Kilroot Ward. How could I go from taking the laces from my shoes and preparing to do an irreversible act to now being given almost full independence in the Kilroot Ward, all in the space of a week? The answer is, though I didn't fully know it at the time, that following that event, a light was shone down a path that I simply didn't know existed – a path of hope.

The following day, at the end of the YAP, the coordinator sat down to speak with me. She was satisfied with the progress I'd made since my introduction into the programme. She believed the tools and resources I'd been exposed to in the YAP, and the sessions I'd done with my psychologist, now needed to be put to the test. She was of the opinion that it was time I was given leave.

My immediate thought was that I wasn't ready. However, the coordinator highlighted the armoury I'd built up in the hospital – mindfulness, deep breathing, exercise and talking were just some of the strategies and coping mechanisms I had in my mental health toolbox, at my disposal whenever they were needed.

I trusted in the confidence that the coordinator so clearly had in me, and was happy for her to put in the request to my doctor, who she was meeting later that day. That evening, I got word back that the request was granted – I had been given three days' leave for the coming weekend. It was a sign of the progress I had made, and something I was proud of.

The time had come. It was Saturday, 31 May, and I was on the way home for the first time in a little over six weeks. Of course, things were going to be different. That was evident as I left the hospital with my mam and Stephanie, as I fully reclined the front seat, put my hood up and pulled the strings on it to the point that all I could see was the ceiling of the car.

Prior to my admission, this sort of thing would have been questioned, but they knew that this kept my mind at ease during my travels now, so an eyelid didn't flicker.

Arriving home, I continued to and through the front door with my hood up and strings pulled. I had no intention of meeting with friends or even being seen in my local area. All I wanted was to be around my family. I settled into the sitting room with my dad right by my side, as we watched the selection of Premier League games that were on offer that day.

This day had an extra significance too – it was my sister Mairead's birthday. She was having a small get-together in the house that evening with some close friends and family. As my dad and I finished watching the football, my mam and Stephanie were putting the final touches on the birthday-decorated house. Mairead, who lived in Swords, was due over shortly along with Colin.

My mind was exhausted, having spent the first part of my time at home focusing on staying in the present, something I'd worked hard on with my psychologist. I went upstairs to have a nap. Although I didn't want to be among the party for too long, as I felt it would be too much for me, I had asked my mam to wake me for the giving of the cake. I was awoken a short while later.

I was nervous making my way down the stairs, approaching the chatter of people in the kitchen – people I hadn't seen since my admission. I quietly walked into the kitchen, placing myself at the back of the group gathered around Mairead as she was given her cake. She blew out her candles, and people went up to congratulate her. Appearing from the back of the group, I sheepishly approached her and embraced her, wishing her a happy birthday. I headed over to the kettle to make a cup of tea before going back upstairs. As I waited for the kettle to boil, my dad's best friend Leo patted me on the back, saying, 'Great to see you,' before returning to the party. The gesture meant a lot to me, giving me a sense of belonging.

The next day, my mam, Stephanie and I were planning to travel to Semple Stadium in Thurles to watch Tipperary and Limerick play a Munster Championship game. I spent most of the morning visualising various scenarios that might arise during the course of the day – from the journey to the stadium to the game itself and the journey home. I had practised visualisation for several years, well before my admission to hospital. That was in a sporting context, however. I used to role play different scenarios that might arise in a game, so that when they did occur, I'd be able to act out the appropriate action in a calm, relaxed manner, having seen it already. This was similar to what I was doing this morning.

The time came to make our way to Thurles for the game. I took my by-now-familiar reclined, front seat position. I engaged in as much conversation as I could for the first portion of the journey. Of course, with it being a long journey, there would be periods of silence, and silence meant an opportunity for ruminating. I prepared for this too. I connected my phone to the speaker in the car and put on one of my favourite comedians, Dara Ó Briain. This not only occupied my mind, but the humour in it naturally lifted my mood. It was a coping mechanism I had picked up from one of the other patients in the hospital. I had originally started doing it to help me with sleep. Having something playing in the background stemmed the hundreds of thoughts that wanted to engulf my mind at night.

We arrived to the ground without any hiccups. You're probably wondering, how was I going to cope with the thousands of people around me at the game, if I wasn't able to sit upright in the car for fear of someone I knew seeing me? I felt the likelihood of running into someone who knew me was very slim, with us being so far out west. Going into the ground, I did feel quite overwhelmed. I felt okay, however, as we took our place in the stands, minutes before the game was due to start.

The game began, and throughout I set myself tasks to keep my mind in check. The game was a distraction in itself, but I felt that there was still an opportunity for my mind to wander. Looking at specifics would mean I had to concentrate that bit harder, distracting my mind further. I broke the game into quarters. In the first quarter, I looked at Tipperary's conversion rate. In the second, I looked at Limerick's conversion rate. In the third quarter, I analysed Tipperary's forward movement; and I compared it with Limerick's in the last quarter. This all served me well, as I managed to stay in the present throughout the entire game. For the journey home I didn't change anything, recognising the success of what I had done on the way to the game. Back at home that evening, I was exhausted but proud of having overcome every potential obstacle I faced that day.

The final thing planned before my return to the hospital came the next day, when Stephanie and I took a trip up to Belfast to see the Titanic museum. The journey to and from Belfast was similar to the one the previous day. The way I was coping may have been slightly out of the norm, but I was okay with that. I was finding a way to cope and didn't care too much how I was doing it. I returned to the hospital that evening, invigorated. The glint of light I had seen only weeks before shone that bit brighter as I reflected, now back sitting on my bed in the hospital, on the success of the last few days.

On Wednesday, 4 June, just under two months after giving my sister Michelle a farewell embrace at the airport in Stockholm, convinced it would be the very last I'd have with her, I was once again in her arms. She had come off the plane that morning, keen to see me. I vividly remember the moment she arrived. I was sitting up on my bed with my headphones on. The curtains were drawn so that I could have full view of the stairs, directly in my eye line about twenty metres away.

My mam and Mairead appeared at the top of the stairs, followed shortly by Stephanie and Michelle. Turning right, they saw me already up from my bed to meet them on their way into the ward. My mam and Mairead parted way to make room for Michelle, who emerged from behind them. We embraced, and I managed to hold it together a bit better than Michelle – having broken from the embrace, I noticed a few tears stream down her cheek.

I showed her over to my room as everyone gathered round. Apart from the telling tears, I could feel the happiness exuding from Michelle, naturally delighted to be reunited with her 'little' brother. I, of course, felt similar emotion toward her. We sat around for a while chatting before leaving the hospital for a couple of hours. Michelle was exposed for the first time to what everyone else had become accustomed to – myself with the hood up, strings pulled and seat reclined. She didn't pass comment at the time, but later recalled that she found it 'worrying'.

It probably won't come as a surprise that we ended up in the Pheonix Park. I wanted to show Michelle the 'sanctuary' that was pivotal in my recovery, particularly in the beginning. I described to her what sort of training I was doing there almost every day and what it did for me mentally, even showing her the one-hundred-metre mark that I had labelled my 'turf' nearly six weeks before.

We spent some more time there, with my mam, Stephanie and Mairead leaving Michelle and I to roam the pitch and have time to ourselves. It was time I was very grateful to have with her. I was dropped back to the hospital, and embraced Michelle once more, saying my goodbyes. This time though, there was no finality to the goodbye, unlike the last time in Stockholm.

It came to the end of that week, and my mind continued to become clearer. I was now able to give thought to a life after hospital. I by no means thought that I had overcome my adversity. In fact, I was aware that depression was something that I may have to live with for the rest of my life. This meant that I was inevitably going to face some bad days. At these points I wanted something tangible to act as a reminder of what I'd achieved in time gone by. This was where the idea of a tattoo was born.

In the beginning, I randomly scrolled through Google images, having searched for 'tattoos for mental health'. Nothing stood out; I needed to be more specific. I tried something different, searching for 'tattoos for depression'. It took a couple of seconds to load before the images appeared in front of me again. The image that I fixed my gaze on immediately was the semicolon. I didn't quite understand what a semicolon had to do with depression though. I investigated further, eventually finding the meaning behind it, and it couldn't have been more fitting. As Project Semicolon put it: 'A semicolon is used when an author could've chosen to end their sentence, but chose not to. The author is you and the sentence is your life.' I shared the idea with my family that evening, as I returned home for my second weekend of leave. They were all hugely supportive of the idea. I wanted to wait until I was discharged from the hospital before getting the tattoo, and this was what I did.

There was one thing I wanted to do in particular on my second weekend of leave. This was to revisit Howth, specifically the cliff walk, as I hadn't been there since the morning of the Leinster U21 final. So, Mairead and

I set out on Saturday, 7 June, to take the exact route we had taken months previously. This was inevitably going to bring up very vivid memories, and perhaps strong feelings as well, but I felt more than prepared for it.

The first thing I noted was the contrast in the weather. This warm, sunny June day was a far cry from the rainy, bleak April weather of our previous visit. This change echoed how I was feeling too. In April, my mind had been dark and bleak, while now, in June, I felt warmth inside. My thoughts were clearer than they had felt for a long time.

The last time we had been here, I recall my gaze hardly lifting from the ground beneath me. Things were different now – my head was up, scanning all around me, taking in the stunning beauty that Howth has to offer. I remarked to Mairead 'how beautiful nature really is'. The remark brought Mairead to a standstill. She turned to face me, smiling and saying, 'Who are you? And what have you done with my brother?' She was, of course, joking, though there was an element of truth beneath what she was asking. My family often used to joke in the past that I should 'broaden my horizons', that there was 'more to life than football'. I never paid any heed to this; for me, the single most important thing in my life had always been football. I guess that at times of adversity, you can find a new respect for the smaller things in life.

As we walked along, Mairead and I reflected on how far I had come since that dark day in April. We returned to the car and I vividly recalled the moment back in April when, as I shut the car door, hundreds of harrowing thoughts flooded into my mind. On this day, I sat into the car and paused for a moment before reaching for the handle on the door. As the door closed, I waited a few seconds before smiling from ear to ear. My mind was clear. I couldn't have ended the trip on a better note than that.

Having returned to the hospital the following evening, I was facing into another week of psychology sessions, meetings with my doctor and the YAP. The week progressed well, building upon my 'mental health toolbox'. I encountered situations that week that I would have found difficult to deal with in time gone past – feeling anxious or depressed, or multiple emotions running through my head at the once. Now though, with the tools and resources I had been developing, I faced these obstacles head on and overcame them.

I was looking forward to going home for my third weekend's leave. My dad came to collect me on the Friday afternoon, and we decided to go for food before going home. I wasn't fussed about where we ate, and it came as no surprise that my dad chose The Avenue in Maynooth. For years, it had been his favourite restaurant, solely for the wings they have. At the restaurant, our conversation very quickly turned to football. I was unaware of how the club or county teams were doing, as I had distanced myself from any social media or television since my hospital admission. Now my dad filled me in on how both were doing.

My relationship with my dad has always been a healthy one. Through no fault of either of us though, our relationship always seemed to be centred on sport. Neither of us was conscious of this. I know I certainly wasn't, because for a large portion of my nineteen-year existence, sport was the only thing I identified with. That was until my admission into St Pat's. I was slowly coming around to the idea that life had more to offer than sport. Now I wanted to broaden my relationship with my dad.

My dad was mid-sentence, talking about all things sport, when I cut across him. 'Do you remember back in the Secure Unit, when you were telling us about what your life was like in East Wall? Tell me more about that,' I said. My dad looked at me, surprised, pausing for a moment before he said, 'Oh, okay then.' Over the next couple of hours, because my dad is hard to stop in his tracks when he gets talking, I heard stories that I'd never heard from him before – nothing to do with sport, purely about my dad and his life. It showed me how closed-minded I had been before, and how little I really knew about my dad and the world that exists outside of sport.

After enjoying another successful weekend at home, I went back to the hospital to continue with my treatment. The cloudiness in my head had got less and less over the last few weeks. Everything was going in the right direction, it seemed. I wasn't so naive to think that all the adversity I'd faced over a two-year period had been dealt with in less than nine weeks, however. Sure enough, on the Wednesday of this week if I recall correctly, the dark clouds began to form once more. I had endured quite a heavy timetable of therapy in these last few days – therapy that involved a huge amount of mental endurance, often leaving me wiped out for hours after a session.

I had been involved in the YAP on Wednesday morning, participating in a group discussion where I offered my voice for large portions of the time. Following that, I'd seen the psychologist, and of course more talking was involved there. I didn't visit the Pheonix Park on this day either, though the physical release would probably have been very helpful. Then, as I attempted to settle into the evening, lying up on the bed with my laptop open, my mind drifted from the present. I began ruminating about situations that led to my current predicament, situations that I've kept private between the nurses, my psychologist and myself up to this present day. Because of the work I'd done with the psychologist, I recognised now that my thoughts were drifting, going off in a spiral. I knew that if I didn't deal with this pattern early enough, it would go beyond repair. The last thing I wanted to do was engage in yet more talk therapy; I was exhausted from all I had done that day. I had to dig deeper into my mental health toolbox.

The tool I chose was to write my thoughts down. I reached for the notebook and pen that I kept in my bedside locker, and began to write down, in an unstructured manner, the thoughts that were streaming through my mind. When my mind began to slow, I pieced together all the thoughts I'd written down. I found that this allowed these thoughts and emotions to become clearer, bringing everything to the surface and in turn bringing light to the situation. I had never really tried this coping mechanism before, but I found it hugely beneficial on this particular evening. I was happy to see this as an indication of the progress I'd made up to this point.

When I wasn't tirelessly running around the Pheonix Park, another place I quite often visited during my time in St Pat's was the Glenroyal Hotel in Maynooth. I was an avid swimmer in my younger years, and it gave me a fairly similar release to the one I got from running. I liked it there too; it was a relatively quiet facility, where nobody knew me.

That was up until this Monday afternoon, 28 June. I had finished my swim, and was just about ready to go on my way when I felt a hand on my shoulder. I turned, immediately recognising the six-foot-plus figure standing in front of me. It was an opposition player that I had had many great battles with already in my short inter-county career. I hadn't had any encounters with anyone outside of the people who visited me in hospital up to that point, so naturally it took me a few moments to gather my senses.

He asked how I was and what had brought me there. My answer was impulsive but honest. I told him I'd been going to the pool there since my admission to hospital and that it helped in my overall recovery. I was on autopilot as I spoke, only realising what I'd said when I stopped speaking. Then I stood, awaiting his response, not quite knowing how it would be received. None of what I had said fazed him; he simply acknowledged what I had said and continuing on the conversation as normal.

A few minutes later, we parted ways. I went out to the car park, where my dad was waiting for me. I didn't tell him about the conversation I'd just had as I reclined the car seat, put my hood up and pulled the strings tight. I reflected on this meeting on the journey back to the hospital, and it brought a smile to my face – not only because of how I had dealt with the whole situation, but how open and honest I had been. The stigma that I had attached to mental health up to only a couple of months before was now gone as far as I was concerned. I believed now that it was something I could cope with in the outside world.

The day of all days, one I'll never forget, came about a week later, on Tuesday, 1 July. I had come off another successful weekend's leave, which gave me another glimpse of how life could be in the future. I had a meeting with my doctor on this Tuesday afternoon, and I filled him in on events since our last encounter. I wasn't expecting what he came out with then. He wrote down the last of his notes, slowly closed over his folder and placed it down on the table to the right of him. He looked steadily over at me and said with a smile, 'I think you're ready to go home, Shane.'

I smiled passively back at him, taking a moment to process what he had said. The word 'home' kept replaying in my mind, as if I was unable to make sense of the whole sentence he had said. A few moments passed before I fully recognised what had been said to me. 'I think you're ready to go home,' I said internally, lifting my head to meet the doctor's gaze. 'Seriously?' I smiled broadly at my doctor, and he nodded. Multiple thoughts and emotions were flooding through my body. But these emotions were of a positive nature. My doctor began to discuss the plan for my aftercare, all of which passed right over my head. All I could think of was that I was going home.

Naturally, I couldn't wait to tell my parents, who were both coming to visit that evening. I returned to my room, along the way telling the nurses the news I'd been given. They were, of course, delighted for me. I had some time to spare before the arrival of my parents, and this was when everything began to sink in. I sat up on the bed, put my headphones on and reflected.

My mind vividly took me back through what had been, and still is, an unforgettable eleven weeks. Memories such as my first day, nervously walking into the dining area, not knowing I would meet friends for life; going public with where I was; the Secure Unit; the dark days and nights; the Phoenix Park; the YAP – it was all going through my mind like a slideshow. It was satisfying to consider where I had been less than three months earlier, ready to surrender to life; while now I could see a path ahead, illuminated with hope.

As I sifted through the turbulent memories of this time, I never once had the feeling of 'job done'. It was more like, 'That's a start.' I knew I hadn't won my battle with depression. I knew every day would be a battle, but now I had the tools and resources to deal with it.

My parents arrived, and sat at my bedside. I remember that I couldn't stop smiling as they sat, looking at me. 'I have some good news,' I began, pausing for a moment to create some suspense. 'I was with my doctor this afternoon, and he told me I'm ready to go home.' I stood up as my dad came over to embrace me. 'I'm proud of you, son,' he said, taking a step back before coming in to embrace me a second time. My mam, not surprisingly, found it hard to keep her emotions in check as I went over to look into her tear-filled eyes and embrace her.

We sat back down, collectively letting out a huge exhale. The brief silence that followed will stick in my memory forever – looking at my parents at the end of the bed, both wearing beaming smiles. Sitting there together, we contacted my three sisters individually to tell them the news – their happiness reverberated through the phone.

The day came – Friday, 4 July 2014, my final day in St Patrick's mental hospital. In the build up to it, more people became aware of my imminent departure – the nurses I'd shared some of my darkest moments with; patients who became lifelong friends; and my two best friends, who gave unconditional support throughout. I was mentally drained from regurgitating the same story to everyone, but sharing the news brought me a deep sense of pride.

Up in my room on this Friday afternoon, having come from my last YAP session, I gathered my belongings from my wardrobe – each item of clothing brought with it a memory from the last eleven weeks. I emptied the bedside locker, holding on to the notepad where many of my emotions were transcribed, particularly in the last few weeks. I gathered up my shoes, recalling the time when they were lace-less.

Stephanie and my dad arrived, and I said my final goodbyes to the patients and nurses on the ward. We went down the two flights of stairs, hung a right and then a left, and walked the long corridor to the exit. A smile spread itself across my face as we arrived at the car, placing my bag into the boot and taking my customary reclined position. The barrier lifted and we made our way home, to what would be a new beginning in life for me.

CHAPTER 6

THE AFTERMATH

My life 'on the outside' began. I'd be lying if I said I wasn't nervous. Although the eleven weeks I had spent in St Pat's had given me the confidence to know I had a foundation on which I could rebuild my life, my integration back into society was naturally going to be slow.

My parents told me of recent conversations they had had with Jim Gavin and with Philip Duffy, my boss at Texaco. Jim had said, 'The door will always be open' for me, if and when I chose to come back. Philip had told my dad that my job 'would always be there'. I had avoided this conversation with my parents while in St Pat's, scared to discover my fate following my admission. I was glad I didn't need to worry about either Jim or Philip. Their responses to the situation I found myself in really showed the measure of these two men.

I felt I needed more time to ease back into society before deciding to rejoin the panel and making a return to work. I kept everything low-key, spending most of my time with my family and working on my mental health each day, utilising the tools I'd picked up in St Patrick's. I used an app called Headspace as part of my morning routine, setting me up for the day ahead. This brings you through guided meditation and mindfulness sessions lasting about ten minutes. I was layering on to what I'd learned in hospital.

Around mid-July, I decided to reintegrate with my friends. There was a barbeque planned one summer evening. Karl and Moe had told me about it the week before, and I decided it would be a perfect opportunity to link back in with everyone.

The morning of the barbeque, I began with my ten-minute meditation, now part of my daily self-care. In the afternoon, I went for lunch with Stephanie and Mairead in the Avenue in Maynooth, a place I had fond memories of with my dad. We went home after this and I got ready to meet up with my friends that evening.

My mind was in a good place prior to heading up to Niall's house, where the barbeque was. There were, of course, some butterflies in my stomach as I drove up to the house. I parked up and took a few deep breaths in the car before walking up the driveway and ringing the doorbell. Niall's parents both answered, greeting me by way of a hug and saying, 'Great to see you again.' They showed me out to the back garden where my friends were, along with a delicious smell of meat being cooked.

I didn't quite know how my friends were going to react, having not seen me since before my admission. As I appeared, I heard a collective, 'Ah, Shane, good to see you, pal.' I made my way around the table, saying my hellos, with a few standing up to give me an embrace. I found a seat at the top of the table, between Mark and Niall. I sensed they were a bit hesitant, unsure of how to broach a conversation with me. So I asked them what they had been up to over the summer, going on to talk about football and life in general.

I was comfortable with my surroundings in the beginning, but when conversation began to open up to the wider table, I began to retreat into my shell. I was confident to engage in one-on-one conversation, but wasn't quite there with interacting in a larger group. My mind began to slip away from the present, with the voices around me now sounding more like 'murmurs'. I began to feel self-conscious and anxious.

My urge was to get up and leave the table, and in times gone past, I would have done just that. Now though, I used a skill I had picked up in hospital – opposite action. Here I was, in a situation where I felt anxious. My instinct was to avoid the situation. However, I had learned that when we avoid, we don't learn that the situation is not dangerous, so we continue to feel anxious should a similar situation arise again. The only way to change how we feel is to learn that the situation is not dangerous, by doing the opposite of what we feel like doing. So, I assessed why I was feeling anxious.

The reason for my anxiety was that I thought people might be noticing that I wasn't engaging in the conversation. But when I looked around at the reality, it was very different. My friends were focused on themselves and the conversation going on around the table. I stayed at the table, brought myself back to the present and engaged in conversation with Mark, who was still sitting beside me. My anxiety diminished with each passing minute. A short while later, I decided it was time to return home, proud of the obstacles I had overcome but exhausted from the few hours I had spent with my friends.

The work I'd done with my psychologist in St Patrick's was only the beginning. My integration back into society would include sessions with a new psychologist, to continue the work. The Gaelic Players Association (GPA) was hugely helpful in helping to source one. They had contact with a very well-known and sought-after psychologist by the name of Joe Griffin, based in Athy, County Kildare. Joe had had players sent to him by the GPA before, and had built a reputation for himself as one of the best around.

My first encounter with him was around mid-July. As my dad and I made the trip from Dublin to Kildare, the thought at the forefront of my mind was, 'I hope we're on the same wavelength.' I knew of patients in St Pat's who, for one reason or another, unfortunately didn't strike a chord with their psychologist, making it difficult to make real headway. I was lucky not to have had such issues yet, immediately hitting it off with mine. I hoped I would be as lucky this time around. As we drove up the cobblestone driveway, my heart rate rose rapidly, along with the doubts in my head. As the car came to a stop, my dad reassured me that everything would be okay.

I made n.y way around to the side of Joe's house and rang the bell. There was the sound of a dog barking, then footsteps approaching the door. The door opened and Joe extended his hand and introduced himself. His office had a book shelf covering one wall, where Joe's seat was. On the opposite side of the room was a green recliner, very comfortable! Directly behind this was a window looking out to Joe's garden and the barking dog I had heard. Joe's welcoming smile and manner put me at ease straight away.

Our session began and within a few minutes I knew I had got lucky for a second time, immediately striking a chord with Joe. His approach was going to be slightly different to the psychologist in the hospital. He got me to go right back to the very beginning of when it all started for me, and from there to the present day. The session ended after an hour and I returned to the car mentally drained.

During our journey home, I asked my dad if what I shared with Joe was confidential. I thought for some reason that things may have been different to the hospital. I panicked for ten minutes, while my dad assured me that everything would of course be confidential. Eventually, my mind discontinued the spiral it was going on, and came around to the fact that what I had shared was indeed confidential.

It was natural that I felt like this. After all, Joe was only the second person that I allowed learn of the two years of turmoil I went through. Of course, my closest friends and family were aware of some of the suffering I had experienced, but nobody else got the details I had now shared with two psychologists. Regardless, the next stage of my recovery had begun and I was excited to see what it could do for me.

Having structure was important in my everyday life, and getting back into normal routines of training, working and socialising would allow me to build this structure. It would be a gradual process until I built up enough confidence and courage to have all aspects of my life back up and running. The next thing I reintroduced to my life was work. The environment of Texaco meant that I could build up my confidence with social interactions while serving customers.

The thought of this initially frightened me. I thought it was a step too far at this early stage, but the sooner I faced the fear of engaging with the general public the better. So, towards the end of July, I went down to speak with Philip. I hadn't seen Philip or any of my colleagues since the middle of April. I didn't quite know how they would react to seeing me again, and I wondered, would they treat me differently?

I entered the shop, glancing over at the tills to acknowledge my two colleagues who were on shift. I didn't stop though, but made a beeline toward Philip's office. He wasn't expecting me on any particular day or time, having simply said that I could come down whenever I felt comfortable. I pushed open Philip's door, and he immediately rose from his chair after recognising me. 'Great to see you back,' he said, shaking my hand firmly and offering me a seat beside his desk. We engaged in some small talk before I said I was ready to come back, if he'd have me. 'Of course, we'd love to have you back,' he said without a moment's hesitation.

A few days later, I was placed back on the roster and my first day back was imminent. Now I had to keep my mind from thinking irrationally about the whole process. I managed to do this and before I knew it, I was walking into work, about to face my first day back.

It was only then, when I made my way behind the till to approach my colleague Paul, that panic slightly set in. 'What will he think? What will he think?' I worried repeatedly. I needn't have worried. We shook hands and as we stood back, Paul said, 'Great to have you back, my man'. This relaxed welcome made those first few days back at work that bit easier than they could have been.

This last month of my life was very different to how I had been living before being admitted into hospital. Ten minutes of meditation and mindfulness each morning set me up for the day ahead. I was seeing a psychologist on a weekly basis. I was taking medication on a daily basis. I spoke openly and honestly with my family when I didn't feel quite right, and the times I didn't feel like talking, I wrote things down. I was back socialising with my friends, but with a different state of mind. I had begun working again, which gave me a platform to develop my interpersonal skills. These things all had one thing in common – they all positively benefited my mental health.

One other aspect of my life that certainly brought me to a better place mentally was sport. Throughout my time in hospital, I managed to keep myself physically fit with countless trips to the Phoenix Park and the occasional swim at the Glenroyal hotel. I had continued in this vein since leaving hospital, but there was something missing – a team environment. I knew the bodily sensations that I had felt meeting back up with my friends and returning to work were going to come up again rejoining the Dublin senior team, but the love that I have for the game trumped my concerns.

Towards the end of July, I made my return to the squad. I met up with Jim in the Portmarnock Golf Links hotel a few days prior to my first session back. He laid things out plain and simple: the likelihood of me playing was less than for other players, as I had been away for so long. But if I had the hunger to push myself up the pecking order, adding something to the group along the way, then he was more than willing to accept me back into the squad. This made complete sense to me, and my return to the squad was official.

My first session back was a gym session out in our base in Blanchardstown. Naturally, thoughts were swirling around in my head in the lead up to it. I tried to take confidence from how I had handled meeting up with my friends and returning to work, but I knew that this was very different. It would be intimidating for any nineteen-year-old to walk into a dressing room of thirty men, especially men of the stature of the Dublin senior football team. Added to that, I had a label over my head that created additional anxiety for me.

I tried my level best during the journey from Portmarnock to Blanchardstown to steer my mind away from any irrational thoughts that were hanging over me. I had my music on in the car that reminded me of happy times, and I made sure to maintain control of my breathing as I went. Both of these helped, and I soon found myself parked up outside the training ground.

I had arrived in good time, and as I made my way into the dressing room to drop my gear bag in, I didn't see any of my teammates along the way. This added slightly to my apprehension. The first person who appeared was our strength and conditioning coach, Martin, who came over to me as I was stretching at the warm up area. I stood up as he shook my hand firmly, saying, 'Welcome back.'

Apart from being one of the best strength and conditioning coaches around, Martin is an even better person. He has time for everyone, taking a genuine interest in not only the player but the person too, and he oozes an aura of confidence that is contagious. We spoke for some time as my teammates began to arrive, each one of them welcoming me back as they came in. Martin left and I continued with my warm up. Paul Flynn approached me from behind, patted me on the back and, staring directly at me, put his thumb up and nodded. Paul's gesture really had an effect on me, giving me that extra bit of confidence I was searching for to really engage with the squad in the session, and those that followed.

A little over a month after leaving the hospital, I decided the time was right to get the semicolon tattoo. I had been drawing the semicolon on my wrist, just below the palm of hand. There was a reason for why I chose this spot on my body: oftentimes when someone is upset or crying, their hands go straight to their face. I knew I was going to have my good and bad days, as everyone does, so I wanted the semicolon to be in my line of vision as my hands went up to cover my face. I hoped it would act as a reminder that no matter what I was going through, it would pass.

My mam and Stephanie came with me to Swords Ink to get the tattoo. I remember explaining the reasoning behind it to the tattoo artist. His eyes were fixed on his desk, concentrating on drawing the stencil. As I explained what it represented, his head slowly rose from the page to look at me, dropping what he was doing and reaching out his fist in a sign of respect. I stayed mute as the tattoo was drawn on, reflecting on times gone by and smiling.

My return to the Dublin squad lasted all but a month. On 31 August, Donegal defeated us in the All Ireland semi-final on a score line of 3-14 to 0-17. During my short time back, I hadn't managed to break into the match-day squad. I did manage, however, to prove that I was more than capable of coping within a team environment again. It was a small victory in what was overall a disappointing way to end the Championship campaign.

The following month saw me take up a place in DCU, studying Sport Science and Health. Two men who were hugely influential in making this happen were Michael Kennedy and Professor Niall Moyna. I hadn't seen Niall since August the previous year, and neither he nor I could have foreseen the journey I'd go on in that time. Michael, being part of Jim's management team, had seen me make my return to the squad and was excited at the prospect of me beginning my undergraduate degree in DCU.

Niall, who is head of the School of Health and Human Performance, and Michael, who was head of Gaelic games, wanted to put measures in place to make my transition into third level as comfortable as possible for me. So, the week prior to the commencement of freshers' week, they invited me in to talk through what was available to me during my time in college. Niall started off by letting me know that his door was 'open at any time of the day' if I had any issues or concerns. One of his PhD students, Sinead, was available to give me grinds in any subject I found difficulty in. I knew Sinead, having already received grinds off her in the lead up to my Leaving Certificate. Again, that was through the helping hand of Michael, who I had met in the January of sixth year, when I was drafted into the senior team. Michael echoed what Niall had said – his door was also 'always open' if I ever needed him. In addition, Michael handed me the key to an unoccupied room around the corner from his office. He told me I had free use of it if I wanted to escape the 'busyness' of the college scene.

As the meeting with Niall and Michael came to a close, a rather tall figure approached the table. He wore a blue jumper that read 'DCU Athletics'. He clearly knew who I was, as he said, 'Shane, very nice to meet you. I'm Enda Fitzpatrick.' I was struck by how penetrating his voice was. He didn't hang around too long, but told me to 'approach' him should I need anything.

I went away from the meeting with an overwhelming sense of gratitude. I couldn't get over the lengths Niall and Michael and others were willing to go to, simply to make my time in DCU as stress-free as possible.

I managed to get through freshers' week unscathed. In truth, I showed up on the first day to receive my timetable and listen to some of the lecturers speak for a few hours before heading off home. College began on the following Monday.

My first lecture was in the Terence Larkin Theatre, a tiered lecture room with the seats in a 'U' shape. As I recall, the lecture in question was physics. There was a mix of classes, which meant there were a couple of hundred students in the room. I hadn't conversed with anyone in my class yet, with first-day nerves a major reason for this. I was sitting about halfway up the lecture room, directly in the middle of a long row, with ten to fifteen students on either side of me – my first mistake!

Shortly into the lecture, my mind drifted. I began to feel self-conscious with the sheer amount of people surrounding me. My mind went spiralling, with irrational thoughts flooding in: 'Are the group behind laughing at me?' 'Have they noticed I'm sitting uneasily?' Unlike in other recent times, I wasn't able to catch my thoughts and stop the spiral. My immediate instinct was to leave the room, though I knew I would bring attention to myself, and disrupt people sitting either to the left or right of me. I thought, 'If I move fast, less people will notice,' as I nervously reached for my bag, stumbling over the students sitting to the right of me. I kept my head down, eyes fixed to the floor, and made a dash for the exit door.

I hurried out into the open air and toward the Helix theatre, fifty metres away. I located the toilets at the Helix, and locked myself into a cubicle in an effort to regain my composure. A number of minutes passed, taking long, slow breaths followed by controlled breaths out. My breath came back to a manageable level, but I stayed in the cubicle a while longer to be sure I had overcome the worst of it.

I left the toilet and found a seat on the ground floor of the Helix. I texted Sinead, knowing she would be on campus, and asked if she would 'Come to the Helix – I need to talk.' I didn't have to wait long for Sinead to come in through the front door, with worry etched on her face. By this time, my thoughts were at a manageable level, and I calmly explained what had happened. Although I was okay now, I didn't want my mind to wander again, and having Sinead there to talk to was really helpful. After speaking to Sinead, we both decided it was best for me to go home, bringing a premature end to my first day in college. I reflected later on that evening on what had happened. I could easily have seen my first day as a 'failure', but in fact, I decided it was a success, as I had dealt with the situation the best way I could, using the resources I had at hand.

During the latter end of my stay in St Pat's, I voiced my opinion on mental health to my parents, saying more than I would have in the beginning.

One thing I was adamant about was that when I came out of hospital, I wanted to share my experiences with the wider public when the time was right. I had been to one of the worst places a human being could get to in their lives, and I had always said, 'I would never wish it on my worst enemy.' I experienced what the power of talking had done for me and the other lucky patients in St Patrick's, but I knew there were people like me still out there, suffering in silence. I was privileged to be in a position that whatever I said or did in the public eye would be heard further afield than most. I didn't know how, when or where I was going to get my message heard, however. That was until I received a message in late September from an employee on the Sean O'Rourke show at RTÉ Radio 1. They had gotten my number from the chairman of my club, who had asked my dad if it was okay to contact me. After some back and forth between RTÉ and myself, it was confirmed that I would come on to the show to share my story alongside Mayo goalkeeper Rob Hennelly and Colin Regan, former Leitrim footballer and GAA community and health manager.

On Thursday, 9 October, my dad and I made our way out to RTÉ HQ in Donnybrook. I felt quite calm in the car on the way over. It was only when we reached HQ that I began to feel somewhat nervous about the situation I was about to be in. 'Hi, I'm here for the Sean O'Rourke show,' I said to the receptionist, my heart beating a little faster. 'Of course, just take a seat and I'll get someone up to you now,' she said. My Dad acted as a good distraction, engaging in conversation with me as we took our seats.

Before long, we were brought downstairs to the control room – where the sound engineers work as the live radio plays out in the background. I peered beyond the sound engineers, through a large window, to see Sean in the live room conducting the show. As I was taking everything in, Rob and Colin arrived. They both shook my hand before taking seats – quietly, so as not to disrupt the sound engineers. After exchanging a few whispers, the show broke off for an ad break. and an assistant came over to inform us that we were on next.

We went into the live room, being greeted by Sean one by one as we took our seats opposite him. I looked to the right of me, noticing Rob and Colin putting on headphones that were on the desk in front of us. 'Clearly not their first time on air,' I thought as I nervously followed suit. The ads were playing out in the background as Sean said, 'I'll be coming to you first, Shane.' The introduction music came in immediately following this. I swallowed the lump in my throat and prepared myself for the questions that were coming.

It was all a bit of a blur from that point on. I spoke as openly and honestly as I could about my experiences leading up to my hospitalisation, about the time I spent in St Pat's and what life had been like since leaving. I was very aware that this was all being broadcast to listeners around the country, and that my story could potentially help to illuminate a path to recovery for somebody. This thought gave me huge satisfaction as my air time alongside Rob and Colin came to an end. I placed the headphones back down in front of me and took a huge breath out.

My dad and I shared a long embrace as I returned to the control room. I couldn't wipe the smile off my face, especially when Colin told me, 'You're a natural on the airwaves.' I switched my phone off 'airplane mode' and saw that my social media accounts were lighting up: 'fantastic interview', 'courageous', 'brave', 'raw', 'honest' and more and more along these lines.

That evening, I came back to the many messages I'd received throughout the day. I was taken aback by the amount of good will being expressed towards me. Many had resonated with what I had to say; some messengers even shared their own experiences with me. I went to bed that night with warmth inside of me, knowing that I had affected many people in the position I was once in.

I continued to grow as a person as the days and months passed. It came to what many refer to as 'the most wonderful time of year' – Christmas. I vividly remembered how the previous Christmas was for me, when I truly believed that it would be my last. In the present, things couldn't have been more different. I was surrounded by those who witnessed the journey I'd been on, and I was grateful for every single one of them. I was no longer a self-absorbed boy who thought the only thing that mattered in his life was football. I had broader horizons now, and was appreciative of the most simple of things life had to offer. One of those 'simple' things was family. I don't think I ever intentionally neglected my family, but I guess I never reflected on them in the way I did now to fully appreciate what they meant to me.

There was one moment that illustrated the new way I had of thinking and the person I'd become since my admission to hospital. I decided I would buy Christmas cards for everyone that would be there for Christmas dinner – everyone being my family, including Colin and Joey. I spent a couple of hours on Christmas Eve writing out personalised messages in each card, attempting to express what each person meant to me. Obviously, this required me to sit and reflect what each person truly did mean to me before putting it down on paper.

You're probably thinking, 'not such a big deal'. However, it was an indication of how far my mind had come from the tunnel-visioned, self-centred teenager I had been up to that point. The next day, when I gave out these

Christmas cards at the dinner table, the looks of bemusement said it all. There was silence as everyone at the table read the personalised cards to themselves. The silence was broken by Joey as his head slowly rose from the page, saying, 'Okay, what happened to Shane?' Everyone at the table laughed, but beneath the laughter was the realisation that 'what happened' to me was that I had changed and had developed a new appreciation for family, and for life for that matter.

In January 2015, the inter-county season started up again. Things were different in my sporting world to how they were before. I had added to my ten minutes of meditation every morning, deciding to meditate before heading to training too. In team meetings, I sat at the edge of the row, in case I found myself in a situation like the one I had on my first day of college. I only travelled by bus with the senior team to matches. For the college and U21 teams, I travelled to matches by car, usually accompanied by my parents, who continued to travel all around the country to any match I was involved in. The ultimate goal was to feel comfortable going by bus full time, but as it had been a trigger for me in the past, gradual exposure was the course of action I had decided on. Although this was out of the norm, none of the managers or players questioned it. The common consensus was 'whatever makes you feel most comfortable'.

In the early stages of the year, the focus was more on college and U21 football. Our college campaign came to a premature end towards the end of January, as we were knocked out at the quarter-final stage. U21 football took precedence from there, as we fought to regain our All Ireland crown. It started off well, as we defeated Kildare by four points in the Leinster final at the beginning of April, booking our place in the All Ireland semi-final against Tipperary two weeks later.

Two days prior to the semi-final, I celebrated what had now become a significant date in my life – 16 April, one year since my admission into St Patrick's mental hospital. Interestingly, world semicolon day fell on 16 April too – a symbol I'd worn proudly for the last number of months. I didn't want to do anything extravagant for it, but I thought it would be good to acknowledge where I had come from. I invited Karl and Moe over to my house after training to join my family and I for a cup of tea. We sat around in the sitting room, sharing some stories from my time in hospital. It was all very lighthearted, but I consciously soaked in my surroundings, grateful for the people who were around me. They had all been there in my darkest time, which I very much appreciated on this evening.

Two days later we faced Tipperary. Unfortunately, the result didn't go our way, as we lost out on a score line of 0-14 to 0-12. It was bitterly disappointing. I wanted to quickly erase the memory of the match, although this was going to be difficult. My idea to escape the pain of losing was to invite a group of friends over for drinks that evening. However, I hadn't been entirely truthful to the people around me. Yes, I wanted to escape the pain of losing the match, but unknown to everyone concerned, the pain was on a deeper level. I was by no means back in the headspace I'd been in the previous year, far from it. But there were issues going on in my head that I had kept away from my psychologist for some time.

I had been receiving heavy psychological treatment since my admission, treatment that continued with Joe Griffin. It was the most physically and mentally taxing thing I'd ever experienced, facing up to the inner demons that had overpowered me for a long time. I was turning up to appointments with issues swirling in my head, but because of the toll it was taking on me day after day, I pretended everything was okay, reverting back to storing it all up in my head. All this was doing, however, was reigniting the volcano that had lain dormant for some time.

So this particular evening was a disaster waiting to happen. Losing an All Ireland semi-final, repressing my feelings for the last number of weeks and alcohol were simply not a good mix. I thought that alcohol could numb the emotions I was feeling, but instead it had the opposite effect. In the beginning, sitting around with my friends at the kitchen table, the alcohol actually did have the desired effect, lifting my mood. This didn't last long though. Pretty soon, as alcohol can, it revived the memories I had repressed, and my mind went spiralling.

I got up and left the table, heading towards my room down the hall. Karl, who noticed something wasn't quite right, went into the sitting room to my family to make them aware of the situation. During this time, I lay face-down on my bed, as hundreds of thoughts entered my head. From that point, my memory went blank.

What transpired from there has since been recalled by my sister Michelle: 'Joey went in to check on you, noticing that you were face-down on the bed. He came to the side of the bed, at which point you started making grunting noises, quite clearly agitated. Joey, noticing that things weren't right, told Karl, who arrived at the bedroom door, to get everyone out of the house. Within a few minutes, Karl managed to get all of the lads out of the house – they were none the wiser as to what was happening.

'Things intensified as you began to lash out, punching the wall, aggressively biting your hands, trying to hurt yourself. You were incoherent, with a glassy look in your eyes. Joey shouted in to Dad for assistance. Both of them attempted to restrain you by pinning you down, which was a huge struggle as you continued to attempt to lash out at yourself.

'Between all of this, Mam had called for an ambulance. Up until a few minutes prior to the ambulance's arrival, you continued to struggle. Profusely sweating, you eventually calmed down, still unaware though of anything happening around you. The paramedics took no chances, restraining your hands and feet and taking you off in the ambulance. By the time you got to the hospital you were out cold.'

My next memory was waking up the following morning, with my Mam and Stephanie by my bedside. They filled me in on all that had happened. Having been cleared by the psychiatric nurse hours later, I returned home. A few days later, having recovered from the event, I explained what had happened to my psychologist, owning up that I hadn't been entirely truthful. It was certainly a learning experience for me, realising the effect that repressing my emotions could have.

Over the next few months, I was as open and honest as I could be with Joe, my psychologist. It was a hugely difficult period, from May until September. Not only was I working tirelessly with Joe to tackle my inner demons, but I had the added difficulty that that summer of football was plagued with injury.

If you ask any inter-county footballer what time of year they look forward to the most, I guarantee that the vast majority will say the summertime. There is no place quite like Croke Park on a summer's day, packed to the rafters, as you fight for the biggest prize of them all – the Sam Maguire.

I was already dealing with my mental battles before my injury woes began. Although I'd built up many tools and resources to help me, exercise was still my number one outlet, especially football. I was still at every pitch and gym session, but I was off with the physiotherapist doing modified training until I was able to reintegrate into the group sessions. I had experienced injury before, as every athlete has. Looking on at other players in your position, playing week in, week out, and consistently improving is only part of the battle. Over the two years when I'd kept everything within, I had felt I was on the periphery even though I was very much in the thick of it – I was there physically, but mentally I wasn't. Fast-forward to where I was now, I was in a much better headspace, but still feeling on the periphery of things due to my injury.

I did make a return to collective training in the middle of the summer, but it was very short-lived, as I had a repeat of my original injury. This led to me reverting back to my old ways again, bottling everything up inside. I was a ticking timebomb. It wasn't a question of if, but when, my next implosion would be. Sure enough, on the day of all days, it happened.

Sunday, 21 September 2015 – All Ireland final day. Every inter-county footballer aspires to be in Croke Park, on that pitch, vying for the coveted Sam Maguire. I was there, but I was up in the stands, watching on as we overcame Kerry by three points in a rain-soaked battle. I was there for the aftermath too – the celebrations on the pitch, continuing on to the dressing room, and then back at the Gibson hotel where the banquet was held. I tried my utmost to share in the joy of my teammates, but the emotions I had repressed for much of the summer were surfacing and I was in a dangerous place.

The celebrations at the hotel came to an end, and we ventured out into town to continue our revelry. My teammates and I went to a nightclub called Xico. Two of my friends also joined me, Karl and Harry. Neither they nor anyone else were aware of anything untoward from me, as I kept everything stable on the surface. As quickly as the alcohol was going down though, so too was my mood. I can't recall the exact details of the internal dialogue I was having, but I know I kept filling my own head with negative judgements of myself.

At some point late in the night, I quickly became 'agitated', according to Karl. He recognised some of the signs of the panic attack he had seen in my house back in April. Karl recalled the night later, as my mind went blank: 'Me, you and Harry were standing around talking. You'd gone quiet, not offering a voice in the conversation. I knew something was up. You couldn't stand still, eyes wandering and aggressively pulling at your clothes. It was then, without saying anything, you turned and made a beeline toward the exit. Harry was unaware of what was happening, and looked to me in wonderment as I told him, "We have to go," following behind you.

'Halfway up the stairs to the exit, you smashed a bottle on the ground. Upon reaching the exit, you burst by two bouncers who were on the way down to see what the commotion was. You'd gone twenty metres down the street, at which point we caught up on you. I tried to get your attention, asking was everything okay, but you were incoherent, pacing up and down in the same spot and muttering to yourself, scratching aggressively at your head. Within a split second, you started hitting out at a shop that was metres from us, at which point I called back down the street for help as you started to lash out on yourself. Everything was reminiscent of that night in April.

'We got you to the ground, as you continued to try to hurt yourself. At this stage, a few teammates and onlookers came over to help restrain you, and an ambulance was called. Not too long after, it arrived and I came with you to the hospital. I contacted your sister, who came a while later along with your parents to the hospital.'

Almost like déjà vu, my next memory is waking up in the hospital. As I was gathering my senses, I peered down at my hands, both with bloodied and bruised knuckles. I let out a sigh, as if to say 'not again'. I was embarrassed as my parents came to my bedside, ashamed to even look them in the eye. There wasn't a lot said between my parents and I at the hospital, or even when I returned home that evening. It was only in the days that followed they told me what Karl had said to them.

I worked alongside Joe in the month following my panic attack, dealing with the issues that had surfaced in recent months as well as continuing with the ones that had built up over a longer period. Towards the end of October, Joe advised me that it might be time for some change. He felt the work he had done with me was coming to an end, and that a different approach would help me further. I had grown close to Joe since the first time I met him. He had given me tools and resources that allowed me to cope. Of course, there were a few hiccups on the way, but that was to be expected. 'I've given you all the tools and resources I have to offer. It's now time to add something new in there,' he said.

It wasn't as if he was leaving me at the side of the road – far from it. He had spoken with the GPA about the change he was proposing. They had decided that the best man for the next step was Dr Francis Valloor, a clinical psychologist with over twenty-five years' professional experience in psychotherapy, training and supervision, assessment and spirituality. I thanked Joe for everything he had done, and a few days later, at the beginning of November, I had an appointment to see Dr Francis.

My first encounter with Dr Francis was on 6 November 2015. Much like with Joe and the psychologist back in St Pat's, I was hugely apprehensive about meeting him. The same questions entered my mind as I made my way up the driveway to his office, attached to the side of his house: 'What if he doesn't relate to me?' 'What if? What if?' When he answered the door, I peered up to take in a grey-haired, well-dressed Indian man wearing glasses. He extended his arm to greet me, and ushered me in to my seat. The room was extremely small, with cream-painted walls, with shelves of books and a desk. There was a locker to the right of me as I sat down; on it stood a clock, two glasses and a jug of water.

Dr Francis began to speak, and his soft voice put me at ease within a few minutes. Our first session lasted an hour; within it, he told me of some of the work we would be doing – including EMDR (Eye Movement Desensitisation and Reprocessing), in which he is an expert practitioner with twenty-five years' experience; a body-centred approach to help build my confidence and understand how I embody my emotional stress; examination of my relationship behaviours and who I am; breath, speech, movement and posture work to deal with my patterns of embodiment. All of this sounded overwhelming, but he assured me that as time went on, I would become more comfortable with these various methods and elicit benefits from them. I went away from my first session intrigued about what the next chapter of my recovery would conjure up.

In the lead up to the New Year, I had the itch to get more tatt os. The semicolon had served as a timely reminder on many occasions, especially in times of difficulty, of how far I had come. In recent times, I had become more comfortable with who I was and the experiences I went through – there were dark and harrowing moments, but they shaped me into the person I am today. I wasn't ashamed to put my 'story' on my body. So, I began to brainstorm; I wanted something with meaning. There were several contenders, including a rose, representing life; a skull, meaning death; a clock, indicating time – I wanted the time to read 3:26, the time I was brought into this Earth; a compass, indicating that I had lost my way in life but navigated myself back on track; and finally, the cover image from Coldplay's single 'Magic' – an image of a dove taking flight. This last piece seemed to carry the most meaning; it was a song I listened to when I was in my deepest and darkest moments, when I couldn't see light at the end of the tunnel. For the duration of this song, however, it brought me to a happier place.

Now that I had my image for a tattoo, the next thing was to choose a tattoo artist. I talked to my cousin, who is covered in tattoos, about my ideas. She recommended a guy named Eddie who has a studio called CrazyCat Tattoos out in Ballyfermot. In two sessions in January and February, Eddie completed the piece. I told Eddie the meaning behind it, and of my mental health struggles, and he was taken aback by how comfortable I was talking about what he said was still a very 'stigmatised' topic.

My life continued in its usual hectic manner. I was juggling an inter-county career, a job, an undergraduate degree and, when I had time, a social life. I made sure I did allow myself some down time. Although keeping busy is one of the best things you can do when dealing with difficulties in your life, it's also important to recognise these difficulties for what they are. I prioritised having fifteen minutes every day just to sit and allow whatever thoughts or emotions that wanted to come into my head, to do so. On some days, I sat in silent meditation, while on others, I used apps such as Headspace to guide my meditation. I had learned that this was important for me; if I neglected this daily practice, it could lead to a build-up of negative emotion.

One day on which I certainly didn't forget to sit with my thoughts was 16 April. I couldn't believe how fast time had gone; it was now two years on from my admission into hospital. It's amazing how when you go through hard times, you appreciate the smallest things in life. I had experienced this over the two years since leaving hospital – from a simple pat on the back to being in the company of loved ones. My two-year anniversary had me feeling appreciative from the moment I got out of bed. The weight of the world I had felt two years before was no longer with me.

The plan to celebrate this fact was to take a trip out to Howth with Mairead. As we sat waiting for Mairead's arrival, my mam and I made time for reflection. I was sitting upright, chest out, bright-eyed and full of conversation, a far cry from the son my mam found in a sorrowful heap, dejected and defeated, on the morning of the Leinster final.

Mairead arrived and we were on our way out to Howth. I soaked in everything as we went, from the cars going by to exercise enthusiasts out enjoying the April sunshine, right down to my ability to peer all around me. We arrived, parked up, went through the old, rusted red gate and set out on our hike.

I didn't speak a whole lot at the beginning, but now it was because I was taking in our surroundings, hearing the crashing of the waves, the feeling of the wind rushing by my ears and the sound of the gravelly path under each step. Mairead and I didn't engage in much conversation for most of the hike. She recalled that 'Little had to be said. Your facial expressions said it all.' She was right too.

Another summer of football approached. I picked up yet another injury, which left me sidelined for a large part of the Championship. This meant I had not only been dealt a physical challenge, but a mental challenge too; a mental challenge that I certainly didn't cope well with the previous summer, culminating in a panic attack on the night of the All Ireland final. I had done a lot of work with my psychologist in the aftermath of all of this. I had learnt from it, and was aware that should I pick another injury – almost an inevitability as a sportsperson – I would need to do things differently.

The natural low that occurs in the beginning stages of an injury was something I had repressed the previous year. This time round, as my rehab began, I voiced any concerns going on in my head, whether to my physiotherapist, teammates, friends, family or psychologist. There were days when I didn't feel like verbalising my emotions, but having learnt that writing things down was a good release valve, I did this. My injury progressively got better, as did my coping skills.

I had also become quite withdrawn from all aspects of my life outside of football the previous summer. This meant that I had a lot of time alone; time to think irrational thoughts, which didn't aid in my physical or mental recovery. I made sure that this wasn't the case this time. I went back to what I know worked for me, which was having a structure. I would sit down and plan my week ahead. I kept up a busy schedule, including work, training and social life. I made sure to have one thing that I could look forward to each day, whether it was coffee with friends, a walk or a trip to the cinema. It was very much a case of getting back to basics, but these basic coping mechanisms keep you afloat in times of difficulty.

When I eventually made my return to full training quite late on in the Championship, I was in a much better headspace than the previous summer. After an epic encounter with Mayo, which had to go to a replay to be decided, we overcame them by the smallest of margins to win back-to-back All Ireland titles. Although I had played no part in the Championship campaign, I'd had my own personal victory, righting the wrong of the previous year and coming away from it all with my head held high.

In the past couple of years I had shared my story sporadically, from coming out publicly with it while in hospital to my first radio interview with Sean O'Rourke and various newspaper interviews. I had seen the impact it had on people, receiving messages of support on social media platforms and even being stopped on the street by strangers to say how my story resonated with them. This all lit a fire in my belly to do more. I was searching for a platform to spread my message of hope further afield.

In late December of 2016, I was given that platform. I received a message on Facebook, inviting me to speak at a 'mental health in sport' talk. After some back and forth, it was confirmed that my first public speaking event would take place in St Kieran's College in Kilkenny on 23 January 2017.

The prospect of sharing my story had me excited and nervous. I was excited to have been given the platform I was searching for, hoping that it would resonate with at least one person in the room on the night. Naturally I was nervous, as it was my first public speaking event. 'What if I go blank and forget what I'm saying?' I asked myself. 'Thirty minutes is a long time to be up there talking.' Nevertheless, I got to work, preparing what I wanted to include in my talk. My parents helped, sharing details on some stories that I wasn't entirely sure on.

I put the points I wanted to include into a timeline: stories in primary school, progressing into secondary school, hiding my inner demons for two years, my time spent in St Patrick's mental hospital and my life thereafter. I went over my speech over and over again, making sure I left no stone unturned. By the time the event came around, I felt I was as prepared as I could be, although I was still experiencing some nerves in the pit of my stomach.

I was supported on the night by family and my then-girlfriend, who'd all travelled down to the event. It was great that my family were all there, as they seen me in my darkest moments. There were about 100 people in attendance, to listen to myself and Cathal McCarron, an inter-county footballer from Tyrone who has had his own battles with mental health. The MC began proceedings, and before I knew it, my talk began. The nerves I had felt subsided within a few minutes, and I began to get into a flow. I closed off the talk with a message I still share today: 'If there's one thing that resonated with you throughout my talk, please take that and spread that message outside these four walls.'

I received rapturous applause as I exhaled deeply. It was an emotional experience for both myself and my family. I felt hugely proud as members of the crowd approached me, congratulating me, saying it 'struck a chord with them'. I was on a 'buzz' leaving St Kieran's College that evening – it left me wanting more.

In the months that followed, I was invited along to a number of clubs and schools around the country to share my story. The same feeling I had got from my talk in St Kieran's College was felt after each talk that followed. From a selfish point of view, I would have loved someone to come in and share their experiences surrounding mental health when I was going through my difficulties. I was blown away in the days following a talk by the messages I received from people who openly admitted they were struggling, but took hope from the message I conveyed to them. That, for me, is worth more than any All Ireland I've won or may go on to win.

My three-year anniversary came around in April. I was in a slightly more extravagant place than where I had been on the previous two years, that place being Dubai. I took plenty of time to reflect on the glamour of Dubai, grateful for the chance to experience it. When you go away to luxurious places, it's very easy to get lost in it all and forget how you got there. I was intensely aware that without the support of my family, friends, everyone at St Patrick's mental hospital, my psychologists and of course the GPA,

I wouldn't have been in the privileged position I found myself in, enjoying one of the most beautiful places on Earth.

Upon my arrival home from Dubai in early May, I was dealt a blow. I received a phone call from Jim Gavin to tell me that I wasn't part of his plans for the upcoming Championship campaign. I was in the kitchen when I got the news. I sat down at the kitchen table and wept for some time, a flood of emotions running through my body. When I had gathered my senses, I let my dad in on the news and gradually, throughout the course of the day, told the rest of my family and close friends.

Of course, the days that followed weren't easy. I had known nothing else since the age of twelve than the drive to be in an inter-county set up. I'm sure people were waiting to take my place, some probably expecting me to turn to drink to mask my problems and cope with it all. I wouldn't have blamed them either, because in times gone by, that's what had happened.

My mental resilience had grown since then though, and I had learned from mistakes of the past. I needed to look at it from a different viewpoint, to steer away from the negative patterns that could easily follow on from receiving news such as this. I decided to take it as a challenge, to return to club football and work on different aspects of my game. Should the opportunity arise again, I'd have full confidence that I worked hard while being away for a short period of time. One thing I had learned since my time in St Pat's was that there is more to life than football. It was and still is a huge part of my life, but giving time to life outside of football is important too.

As the months went by and I was getting more used to being away from the inter-county set up, I gave time to those other aspects of my life. I spent more time with friends, whereas before I had been concerned about the amount of energy I'd expend, and so would opt to sit in and rest at home.

I enjoyed the odd takeaway – again, in times gone past, I would never have gone near one. People who have not experienced the high-octane pressure of an inter-county squad would probably think that it's bizarre how stringent I was. I'm not saying every inter-county player is like me, but I know many of them make their own sacrifices, which are part and parcel of being an inter-county footballer. It was nice to step out of the bubble for the time being and experience some things I had been missing out on. However, I still had a burning desire to get back involved in the Dublin set up, and sooner rather than later.

As the summer went on, I was experiencing some things for the first time, one of which was going to my first ever concert. The band was Coldplay, who on many occasions, through the power of their songs, had helped me escape from the harrowing places my mind went to. On 9 July, I went to see them play in Croke Park, and it was an unforgettable night. It was strange to see the hallowed turf of Croke Park covered up, to allow thousands of music enthusiasts get up close and personal with Coldplay. Myself and my girlfriend at the time watched on from the upper Cusack Stand. It was visually the most stunning thing I've ever experienced. The stage's catwalk was illuminated along the edges, colours changing with each song. The catwalk expanded out into a circle, which throughout the night would transform into a night sky or a simple acoustic stage. Everyone had bands on their wrists that illuminated to the beat, winking as Chris Martin's voice cut through the air like a shard of glass. Songs such as 'Paradise', 'The Scientist', 'Everglow' and of course my favourite song of all, 'Magic', rang out across the energy-filled stadium.

Throughout the night, my mind wandered sometimes. I had powerful visualisations of the times of adversity I'd faced, whether it was in Stockholm, a place where I thought my final moments may very well have been; atop Howth summit, peering out into the night sky, believing the darkness in front of me would be a permanent fixture; or in the confines of the hospital, sitting staring at the laces of my shoes. At times I became emotional; at others I wore a broad smile, remembering just how far I had come.

When the show ended, the stadium seemed to echo the screams of the audience and the sounds of the band. This being their farewell tour, Coldplay were saying goodbye to one chapter in their life, and preparing to embark on another, hoping to make an impact in whatever they got up to next. There were striking parallels in all of this for me, as I bade farewell to the demons of the past and leaped into a new chapter, illuminating hope not only for myself, but perhaps others around me in hearing where I'd come from.

I enjoyed the rest of my summer, and returned to college in late September, for the final year of my undergraduate degree. Quite early on in the college year, I was given some good news. Although it was unrelated to college, it had a positive impact on all aspects of my life, college included. For some time now, I was gradually being weaned off the anti-depressants I had been prescribed in hospital. In a careful and measured way, I had been reducing the medication that had been part of my life for almost three years.

I was never a huge advocate of medication, especially in the beginning. There is a common misconception that when someone is suffering with their mental health, they can simply take some tablets, and that will cure everything. I knew this wasn't the case, right from the very outset, and I was reluctant to take them in the first place. However, I gradually learned that, no, taking medication didn't cure everything, but it certainly could aid recovery. I was used to waking up and reaching over to my bedside locker to take my medication before getting on with my day.

At times when I was away on training camps, sharing a room with teammates, they would ask, 'is that painkillers you're taking?' I would reply that they were my 'happy pills', 'smarties' or 'crazy pills'. My response would raise a few eyebrows, my teammates not sure whether to laugh or not. Jokes such as this were an attempt to put other people around me at ease, because there was always a lot of awkwardness whenever the subject of mental health was raised. Now, in early November, these jokes became redundant, as I officially became medication free. It was another big step in my recovery.

The New Year came, and I was once again drafted into the Dublin team, for the upcoming League campaign. However, my return to the team was very short-lived. Limited game time throughout meant that by the time the League finished up in early April, I was vulnerable to being let go once more. Inevitably, the call from Jim came in the middle of April, letting me know I wasn't in his plans for the Championship campaign again. It was another blow, after I had worked so hard to get back in. However, this was simply the reality that I had to deal with.

I was making huge ongoing strides with regard to my mental health, despite being dropped from the Dublin squad for the second time in less than a year. So much so that on Friday, 18 May 2018, I had my final appointment with Dr Francis. Four years of psychological treatment by various professionals had come to an end. From dealing with the often dark and painful times of the past, to learning how to cope in my everyday life, to now truly living where I was once only surviving, had been a long, hard journey, to put it mildly.

I had known for some time that my sessions with Dr Francis were coming to a close. We had discussed the prospect of my branching out on my own in the prior months, so I had plenty of opportunity to prepare myself. For four years, I had had the crutch of psychologists to help steer me, but now I was being given the wheel. I would be lying if I said I wasn't scared.

Dr Francis had helped to instil a belief in me that I was ready to go on with my life, independent of him or any other psychologist. It was a belief that I had been building upon since my first encounter with the psychologist in St Pat's, whether I knew it or not at the time. It was a strange feeling, shaking Dr Francis's hand for the final time, thanking him for the place he had brought me to. On the journey home, I was determined to continue along the path that all of these professionals had paved for me.

Change was happening all around me. I was no longer part of the Dublin setup; I had recently finished my psychological treatment; and, towards the end of May, I handed in my thesis, marking the completion of my undergraduate degree. In the days following, an opportunity for further change was put before me. Since being let go from the Dublin team, I had spoken with some of my football friends who had, for one reason or another, chosen to go stateside to play football for a summer. It was something I had never considered in the past, due to my commitments with Dublin. I was no longer in that privileged position, which meant the prospect of a summer stateside was now viable. Some friends let it be known to the clubs they represented over in the states that I was interested in going over.

I didn't have to wait long before the phone started to ring and messages were coming in through social media from various clubs spanning the east to west coasts. One club in particular showed a keen interest – Ulster Gaelic Club in San Francisco. I spoke with James McCann, one of their coaches. He told me a bit about the club and its record, about players that had come from overseas to represent them for a summer and about life in general in San Francisco. I was intrigued to know more.

James passed me on to a man who was known as 'Mr Ulster Club', namely Joe Duffy, and we spoke at length on the phone the following day. I found Joe to be very personable. Two days after speaking with him, my mind was made up – I would spend my summer in San Francisco. Once all the formalities were dealt with, getting the all-clear from work and my club, I was set to go. On Sunday, 10 June, my bags were packed and I was on my way to a summer on the US west coast.

My first and lasting impression of San Francisco: cold! Legendary American storyteller Mark Twain once said, 'The coldest winter I ever spent was a summer in San Francisco.' On my first morning, I stood out on my apartment balcony, wearing a couple of layers of clothing and firmly gripping a piping hot coffee. I didn't mind the cold that much, and it was worth it for the view – not too far in the distance were two of San Francisco's most famous landmarks – the iconic Golden Gate Bridge and Alcatraz Island.

I settled in over the next days and weeks, taking in more of the famous landmarks around the city, such as the stunning Twin Peaks, Pier 39, Fisherman's Wharf and Lombard Street. I quickly found the area and its people very welcoming.

Of course, being over there for the summer meant I would need to earn some money. Joe had set me up with a job in construction – an industry I knew nothing about. However, that didn't matter. My job was simply to transport tools and supplies to the men who were qualified to carry out the job at hand. I was also responsible for keeping the general area tidy – I was joined in doing so by a Galway man, Eanna, who was over on a J1 trip. Eanna and the charismatic Cork foreman Jimmy McMullen were the only other English-speaking workers on site, which made for an interesting and amusing dynamic when trying to work together with the non-English-speaking workers. Jimmy treated Eanna and me very well throughout the summer, bringing us out for drinks after work and inviting us over to his house for dinner with his family. Sometimes he would pull us from the site to head out for a few holes on the golf course, which was only five blocks away from where we were working – a laid back job to say the least!

Then there was the reason I got brought over stateside in the first place – football. Within a few days of arriving, I was heading out to Beach Chalet, our training base for the summer, to meet my teammates. At the heart of the team were the local players, most of whom had emigrated from Northern Ireland throughout the years. The rest of the team was made up of summer transfers from Ireland, most of whom came with a bit of pedigree in the Gaelic football world. The standard was very high, and there were other teams around the area of similar capability.

Our games were played out on Treasure Island, an artificial island in San Francisco Bay, and they took place almost every weekend. Here, thousands of miles from home, there was so much to take in – a new area, new people. However, whenever I stood out in Beach Chalet or on Treasure Island with a size five O'Neill's in my hand, I felt completely at home.

There were opportunities at various stages of the summer to do some travelling. I took full advantage of these times, visiting Lake Tahoe for 4 July; Vancouver, where my best friend Moe was now living, at the end of July; and Los Angeles at the start of August for a UFC event.

My time in San Francisco came to an end in early September, but I still had a bit more travelling left to do – the rest of September saw me reunite with my family, this time in Orlando, Florida, to celebrate my mam's sixtieth birthday. The final leg of an unforgettable summer saw me in Miami to celebrate my twenty-fourth birthday and then, to top it all off, heading to a UFC event in Las Vegas with friends from home in early October.

Toward the end of my stay in the US, my mind turned to what I was going to do when I arrived home. I was planning a year out before returning to college to do a master's degree. I would continue to work in my local petrol station, as it gave me flexibility, which I would need throughout my master's. Of course, I was going to stay playing football.

In this year out, the void that would be left by not having any college would have to be filled. I began to think, 'What means something to me?' Inevitably, football was the first thing that came to mind. Then, mental health was next. I thought a little further. I had been doing talks around the country over the last while. Events like this are on at a certain time, in a certain place, and are only available to people within their vicinity. How could I spread my message further afield?

I thought of a blog I had read not too long before. This was the work of Conor Cusack, a former Cork hurler who had previous with depression. The blog was hugely moving, and resonated with me on many levels. I didn't have to travel to Cork to hear Conor's story – I could read it on my phone, in the comfort of my own home. The simplicity of this really struck me. People nowadays are no more than a few clicks of a button away from any information they are looking for. Perhaps I should write a blog? It would reach a wider audience, and people could access it in their own time.

As soon as I returned from the US, I started looking into how to write a blog. I didn't know where to start, so I went to a former work colleague, Liam Murray, for assistance. While working in the petrol station, Liam had got a master's in creative writing and wrote pieces for various newspapers. Liam laid it out plain and simple for me, and offered a hand: 'Write down what you feel is necessary to include, referring to what you speak about in your talks. Send it on to me and I'll have a look at it.'

We agreed that Liam wasn't going to edit everything, as it could come across as too journalistic and lose some of its authenticity. He would read it and make recommendations on what could be added in or left out, and look at the overall flow and structure of it.

I sent my first draft to Liam in the middle of November. He soon got back to me with some proposed changes. At the start of December I sent on my second draft, and this time he didn't have any changes. I reread it numerous times over the next few days, to be sure I had included everything I wanted to say in the piece.

On Wednesday, 19 December 2018, I was ready to publish. I sat with my laptop in front of me on this morning, with the cursor hovering over the 'publish' button. The story I had held within for two years, bringing me to the point of suicidal ideation, was now a click of a button away from being shared with the entire world. An intimidating thought. However, I decided that if my blog could help even one person not to reach the depths of misery and despair I had seen in my life, then sharing my story with the world was going to be worth it.

After a few minutes of hesitation, I clicked 'publish'. I sat back on my chair, exhaling deeply. I posted my blog on Instagram and Twitter. In the hours and days that followed, my phone didn't stop lighting up. I received messages from across the globe, from people in all walks of life, from both young and old. To say I was overwhelmed by the reaction would be a massive understatement. In the coming days and weeks, I appeared on television and radio stations, discussing in further detail what I had shared. I had a deep sense of pride during it all, and I was taken aback by the warmth shown to me by anyone who'd heard my story.

I didn't foresee what was to come from there. It started with being asked to write this book. On 16 January 2019, I was contacted by Michael O'Brien of The O'Brien Press, asking if I'd be interested in coming in for a chat about a possible book project. I was in work when I got the email. My first thought was that the email was spam. Having realised that it was genuine, I looked for the opinions of close family and friends on how best to approach such an offer.

The prospect of releasing a book brought me similar feelings as the idea of the blog had. Of course, this would be a much larger project, not only timewise, but also in terms of giving out much more details of the darkest and most difficult time in my life. However, I was more than willing to write about all of it. On 15 April 2019, Michael and I put pen to paper on an author–publisher agreement, and I embarked on writing the book you are now reading.

Also in January 2019, I was asked to become an ambassador for Pieta House. It was humbling to be asked to work for a charity that, since opening its doors in 2006, has helped over 58,000 people in suicidal distress or engaging in self-harm. In 2018, almost 8,200 people came through their doors, and they managed over 16,000 calls through their twenty-four-hour freephone helpline. These numbers might seem shocking, but it is very a positive development that people are more willing nowadays to seek the help instead of suffering in silence as I did for many years.

I've experienced that willingness of people to speak up firsthand, especially since the release of my blog. While I thought I would only be taking advantage of the flexibility of my workplace from the end of September, with the commencement of my master's, it turned out that I needed it much sooner. The release of my blog sparked public speaking requests from across the country, starting in early January. I was inundated; public speaking was fast becoming a full time job in the early parts of the year.

This brought a new challenge that I hadn't faced before – regurgitating the demons of the past more regularly had the potential to bring up negative emotions, negative emotions that had led to trouble in previous years. Now, any time I detected that my mood state was wavering, I rescheduled upcoming talks to a later date.

I planned things that I knew would be of benefit to my mental health: music, meetings with friends, cinema trips, an occasional meeting with my psychologist and, of course, exercise, particularly football. This last even posed a challenge – for the first time since 2010, I was going to be back training with the club from the early part of the year, having not received a recall to the Dublin squad for the 2019 campaign. However, I had had experience of this, having been let go halfway through both the 2017 and 2018 campaigns.

Just like in those years, I decided to regard it as a challenge, to return to club football and work on various aspects of my game. Should the opportunity arise again, I would have full confidence that I had worked hard while being away from the county side. The club's aim this year was to gain promotion to Division 1, the pinnacle of Dublin club football, a place where we hadn't been since 2003.

By the end of May 2019, I had delivered over fifty talks nationwide, in schools, sports clubs and corporate settings. My public speaking appearances quietened down during the summer months, while football, work and the book took precedence. Of course, I also made time for some social interaction, something that I knew was paramount to my overall mental health. Scheduling was an important part of balancing all of this – knowing where I would be on what day and at what time helped to stem any anxiety that all this frantic activity could have provoked.

From September, I had the added challenge of scheduling in a full-time master's degree, as I took up a place in DCU, studying for an MSc in Management (Business). A typical day in my life now looked like this:

Gym (6–7.30am)

Book (8–9am)

Lectures (9am–1pm)

Book (1–2pm)

Lectures (2–5pm)

Book/assignments (5–7pm)

Training (7.30–9pm).

Often I would also have to factor in a talk anywhere in the country or a shift in work – as you can see, I had a lot on my plate. However, I had an inner desire to make it all work.

My talks were beginning to ramp up again, and some high-profile ones at that. In early October, I was invited to speak at an event called Zeminar. This event could be described as a social enterprise, held to bring all those invested in the development and wellbeing of young people in Ireland to one place. Starting out in 2016, in just three outings they have already welcomed over 45,000 attendees, making it the largest and most inclusive youth gathering ever seen in Ireland.

This event took place in the National Sports Campus. I joined the inspirational Niamh Fitzpatrick and Fiona Brennan on the main stage, each of us having ten minutes to share our story. While the other two speakers were on, I scanned the crowd of over 1,000 people, at times blinded by the massive stage lights. The majority present were teenagers, and I was taken aback by their attentiveness, as they clung to our every last word. The event was further evidence that times are changing – young people are now much more willing to talk about mental health. On this day, I was proud to play a small part in helping them to do so.

November didn't show any let up when it came to my daily schedule. However, there was really only one thing on my mind this month – the promotion playoff final, with the prospect of moving up to Division 1. If potentially being promoted wasn't enough, there was the added impetus of who the opposition were: St Sylvester's, in their own backyard.

The match was played on a typically wet and miserable November's day, which made for difficult viewing. Having been a tight and cagey affair for the most part, we managed to pull away in the final ten minutes of the game, winning out in the end. Away from the obvious joy, there was a great sense of relief above anything else following the final whistle. The common consensus among Gaelic footballers is that achieving something with your club feels that bit more special than with the county team. Now, I'm not for a second demeaning the inter-county scene, or playing down the euphoric feeling of a victory with your county team, but a club win seems to be a little more special somehow. That's exactly what it was on this day.

Celebrations didn't last for too long, due to the busyness of my schedule – while club football was now over, college football had started back. Now the main priority was preparation for the Sigerson Cup, the elite third-level colleges' Gaelic competition, in January. It was a constant battle to try and juggle everything, particularly the talks – I had surpassed the 100 mark for the year by the start of December.

At this stage, I knew something had to give way before the Christmas period had even begun. I was simply running myself into the ground, not only physically but mentally too. People had been saying to me for months when they learned of my busy schedule, 'How do you manage it all? I certainly wouldn't be able to.' It was the competitive streak in me that wanted to keep it all going, to prove to people that I could take on this seemingly insurmountable workload and overcome it. However, one night in December proved just that – it was insurmountable; it was too much, and something had to give.

In the days leading up to this night, I was noticing signs and symptoms that were strikingly similar to the past – social withdrawal, mood fluctuations and negative spirals. I masked it all. These signs and patterns were nowhere near the severity they had been at prior to my admission into St Patrick's; however, they weren't something to be ignored.

My social withdrawal had become a concern for my close friends. I hadn't been in contact with them for a number of months now, with the exception of the odd message, blaming my withdrawal on my hectic schedule. I eventually gave in and agreed to have a night out with them on Saturday, 7 December, which would overlap with my work Christmas party scheduled for that same night. The idea was that I could be highly efficient and kill two birds with one stone.

We started out the night in Gibney's in Malahide, where I met my three close friends Karl, Moe and Philip. Being an avid Manchester United supporter, I made sure we got there in time to get the best seats in the house – the Manchester derby was kicking off at 5.30pm.

All was not right though. It goes back to when we were younger, when my dad would say, 'Anything you do, do it to the best of your ability.' All that I was doing – training, working, writing, public speaking, studying – all had to be done at 110%, or else I simply wasn't satisfied. Doing that day in, day out, had eventually taken its toll on me. I had spent the day inundated with college work, which left me feeling stressed and anxious.

I sat in the pub, by glance moving between the match and my three friends who were conversing to the right of me. I was there physically, but mentally I was elsewhere. My mind wandered to a conversation going on within, asking, 'What is going on for me?' It was very reminiscent of a time in fifth year, sitting on the bus on the way to a game, my mind coming in and out between the conversation in my head and the conversations going on in the bus.

At times I would come back into the present, and I would turn to my friends, pretending to acknowledge the conversation that was going on. I continued like this for the entirety of the match, before having to head off to my work Christmas party. While saying goodbye, Moe asked, 'Everything all right?' to which I replied, 'Yes, all good.' I knew that he could see something wasn't quite right, but he wasn't going to push me for answers there and then.

I hadn't far to go, a five-minute taxi ride to the White Sands hotel in Portmarnock. I knew I wouldn't have the distraction of the match to blame on my withdrawal; I'd have to dust off the infamous mask and put on an acting performance for a few hours at least. My acting skills were obviously a bit rusty, because not too long after my arrival one of my bosses, Louise, Philip's daughter, sensed my distant manner.

Louise reminds me very much of my sister Michelle – strong-willed, outspoken and driven, but always with a softer side too. This wasn't the first time that Louise had picked up on my fluctuating mood, sensing it at times in work and sometimes lending a listening ear when I needed it. That was the case on this particular evening. Without my having to say anything, she told me what I already knew: that I'd taken on too much, placing unnecessary pressure on myself, and it was having a direct impact on my mental health. Something had to give. This conversation kick-started the re-evaluation I would go through in the next few months.

In the days that followed, I went back to basics, back to the foundations. I planned my week; within it I included time speaking with close friends and family, as well as exercise, meditation and time for writing down thoughts and listening to music. All of these were staples of my 'mental health toolbox', but I needed something more. I knew what that something was, but I was reluctant to admit that I needed it.

That something was my psychologist, Dr Francis Valloor. Part of me felt that it would be admitting defeat to go back to him. 'I should be able to handle this on my own,' I told myself. I also worried about what my family and friends would think if they heard I was going back to my psychologist. These were, of course, the old, familiar irrational thoughts. They swirled around and around in my head before I snapped out of the spiral I was sinking into. I eventually gained a little perspective on the situation, deciding to look on as simply going for a 'top up'.

I picked up the phone and made an appointment, attending a few days later. I discussed the things that were on my mind with Dr Francis, and he helped me to unravel the cloudiness that had blinded me for a number of months. My mind became a little clearer, allowing me to relax into the Christmas period and enjoying some much-needed family time.

At the turn of the year, my mind was focused on the Sigerson Cup. I hadn't yet managed to get my hands on a Sigerson medal – the closest I'd come was in 2016, during my undergraduate degree, when we narrowly lost out to UCD in the final. This campaign didn't start out well on a personal level, as I picked up a minor hamstring injury in the lead up to the opening round, against Garda College. Thankfully, we defeated them by two points, and I was available again for selection the very following week, 19 January, to face Queen's University, Belfast. Paddy Christie, former Dublin footballer, was our manager and he placed trust in me, putting me in from the start against Queen's. We came out convincing winners, setting up a semi-final place against UCD just three days later.

All that had been going on for me prior to Christmas hadn't entirely subsided. However, there wasn't long left in the football, so I decided to give that my full attention before tackling what was really the bigger issue. We cruised into the Sigerson Cup final with a fifteen-point win over UCD. Now there was just one more obstacle to overcome – on Wednesday, 29 January, we faced IT Carlow in a bid to become Sigerson Cup champions for the first time since 2015.

I was fortunate to be given a starting place again, lining out in midfield. Matches of this magnitude are often tight and cagey affairs, particularly in the beginning. That's how this occasion was playing out, as we led by only three points at half time. We were able to turn the screw as the second half wore on, coming out seven-point victors. Celebrations ensued and of course, as ever, my parents were there afterwards to share in my obvious delight.

My performances throughout the competition had caught the eye of the new Dublin senior football manager, none other than Dessie Farrell. He recalled me to the squad the day after the Sigerson final.

In early February, having had numerous conversations with both my family and the DCU people, I took the hugely difficult decision to step away from my master's for the time being. The severity of my situation wasn't anywhere near what it had been back in 2014, but subtle signs were telling me something needed to change. Ignoring these signs before had led to all sorts of trouble and I simply wasn't going to let it manifest into something like that again.

My schedule had freed up somewhat. Yet, approaching the end of February, I had already spoken in thirty different locations nationwide. At this stage, I was glad of the decision I'd made at the start of the month, wondering how I could have coped if I hadn't taken that difficult but sensible step. The return on this was noticeable too – heading into training, I had an extra pep in my step; I was more productive in work; my creative writing mind was discovered once more; and my talks were as energised and enthusiastic as they ever were. However, all this was going to be cut short. For a number of months, I had heard of this thing called 'coronavirus', but little did I, or anyone else for that matter, know the devastating impact it would have.

On 29 February, the first case of Covid-19 in Ireland was reported. On 11 March, the World Health Organisation declared that Covid-19 is a pandemic, while Ireland suffered our first death associated with the virus. I remember the following day, sitting with my parents and Stephanie watching RTÉ news, something that was going to be a common occurrence in the months to follow, as Taoiseach Leo Varadkar announced a series of measures including the closure of schools, colleges and childcare facilities.

In the days and weeks that followed, almost all businesses, social venues and educational and sporting facilities and amenities were shut.

While my parents and Stephanie were out of work for the time being, I was fortunate to still have a number of shifts throughout the week, as Texaco lay under the umbrella of an 'essential service'. Work was keeping me occupied for a certain portion of the day at least; everything else in my life came to a complete standstill, which meant there were a lot more hours in the day to fill. It probably wouldn't come as a surprise that exercise was at the forefront of my mind when it came to thinking of how to fill my day. I managed to get my hands on quite a bit of gym equipment from the GAA club gym before its closure, as well as some footballs. I needed to train alone to stay on top of my game while collective training had taken a back seat.

By 27 March, things were a lot worse, as the country went into 'lockdown'. Now people could only able to leave their homes in 'specific circumstances' or for brief exercise, within 2km of their homes. This time reminded me very much of St Pat's – there was little human interaction, and that feeling of being boxed in. I created a timetable, getting my family involved in it too. I explained to them how I framed it – the 'non- .egotiable' stuff went in first, which for me was work; followed by things that you enjoy, which was mostly exercise in my case; and finally, things to stimulate the mind – reading for example.

I've spoken before about the power of scheduling, and the many benefits that stem from it – establishing a routine, reducing stress, feelings of accomplishment and so on. These were some of the buzz words I heard from my family not too long into lockdown.

Even though my eldest sister, Michelle, was thousands of miles away in Stockholm, we got her involved too. We gathered out in the back garden with Michelle perched up on the table, dialling in through FaceTime, and we all went through workouts that I planned. Besides being beneficial to your physical health, group exercise can be of benefit to your mental health as well. There is a lot to be said for human interaction.

I feared the impact this 'lockdown' phase might have on many people's mental health, even in the early stages. The daily coronavirus updates, though necessary, caused a considerable amount of fear, worry and stress amongst people. The lockdown measures, originally meant to be in effect until 12 April, were then extended until 5 May, only further enhancing my fears of the psychological impact they would have. Activities, routines and livelihoods were all heavily impacted, and many people simply didn't have the tools and resources to deal with all of it. There was a sharp increase in levels of loneliness, depression, harmful alcohol and drug use, self-harm and suicidal behaviour. In years gone by, on occasion, I would receive a message through social media from someone, young or old, seeking my guidance on how best to deal with whatever personal demons they were battling. Since the beginning of the pandemic, however, these messages now came in on a daily basis.

Individuals react differently to global events. Some deal with things in a laid-back, light-hearted fashion, while others obsess and fret and magnify the situation. The daily reports of coronavirus cases and deaths from news reports, social media and health organisations meant that people had massive amounts of information to take in. False information and scaremongering was also flying around, greatly adding to the stressful nature of it all.

People with underlying mental health issues were of course going to be more vulnerable, but indeed people with no prior conditions were now coming into this category as well. Not only was there fear associated with contracting the virus, but also fear regarding the effect it would have on livelihoods and national economies.

People needed an outlet. For many, it was getting involved in the infamous Zoom calls, whether with family abroad, friends from home or work colleagues. Never did we appreciate human interaction as much as we now did, albeit in miniature, through a phone or computer screen. The two years of hell I went through taught me to appreciate the little things in life, and now it seemed that many more people were learning that same valuable lesson!

One insight I have gained is that adversity is to be overcome, not passively accepted. There were obstacles along my path, but they gave me opportunities to create alternative paths, all leading me to become a more rounded and resilient person. For almost six years, I have stood proud atop the pedestal many still put me up on, hoping to illuminate a path for others who might see nothing but darkness. If there was ever a time to shine that light, brighter than it has ever been before, it was now.

A number of clubs, schools and businesses nationwide contacted me, asking me to do virtual talks, and I was only too delighted to oblige. I knew from the countless messages I was receiving that people needed to hear the story of someone who has been to the brink and turned their life around. There are people who haven't yet found the courage to speak up, gripped by the tentacles of depression, and it is especially important for them to hear a voice of hope. I'm by no means saying that I'm the best public speaker in the world – far from it. But if even one person who listens to me finds the strength from my story not to take the step that I almost did all those years ago, then that's good enough for me. I continued to do these talks throughout April, and it was rather poignant too that my anniversary fell in the middle all of this – 16 April, six years since my admission to St Patrick's.

In May, the Government published their five-phase 'roadmap', which would see a gradual easing of restrictions throughout the summer months, slowly reopening Ireland's society and economy. Approaching the summer months, the evenings were getting brighter and our future looked to be heading that way too.

I have to admit, it felt strange in the beginning, meeting up with friends who I'd become so accustomed to seeing through a phone or laptop screen. I, and anyone else I spoke to it seemed, had gained an added appreciation for simple human interaction. I found the time I now spent with my friends more meaningful; we would have more engaging conversations, and got that sense of 'I'm here for you', acknowledging the strange and difficult times we were in and were still facing. I don't think we ever took each other's company for granted, but I guess in times of hardship you really reach a deeper appreciation of your fellow human.

The month of June saw a further easing of restrictions. By 29 June, we had gone to 'Phase 3' of the government's roadmap. This phase brought excitement to all sport enthusiasts in particular, as it marked the recommencement of all sports. I loved the physical and mental challenge that individual training had posed over the last number of months, but there's no comparison to being back amongst it with your teammates.

Covid-19 had also meant returning home for many people who had been living abroad. This meant that faces of old were making a return to the club scene across the country, including at our club. It brought me back to my younger days when these players resurfaced, only adding to the special atmosphere that was being felt in clubs across the country. The delayed and reshaped GAA season would see the club Championship recommence at the end of July.

While football was taking precedence, I was still making time for other areas in my life, including time with family and friends. The time I spent with my family was particularly rewarding. During the months of July and August, we planned a hike or cliff walk each week, often making a full day of it, finishing with a takeaway and movie together at home. It sounds like such an ordinary thing to do, but prior to Covid-19, we all led such busy lives, and we let that blind our judgement on what really mattered – that being, of course, each other. Amongst all the negative that the coronavirus has brought, this realisation was certainly a silver lining.

September came, and all the excitement that football had brought over the past few months came crashing down as we were dumped out at the semi-final stage of the Championship. It was a double whammy, because not only did I have to deal with the disappointment of the club season coming to a devastating end, but I'd learnt that my inter-county aspirations weren't going to come to fruition when it all kicked back off in mid-October: I had not been recalled to the Championship squad.

Meanwhile, Covid-19 cases were increasing again throughout September, culminating in whispers by the end of September that a second lockdown was on the horizon. On 19 October, this fear was realised when the Government agreed to move the country to Level 5 lockdown for six weeks, until 1 December.

Personally, I wasn't fearful of the second lockdown. My fear lay externally, just as it did in lockdown one – fear for the wider public. People were not being armed with the tools and resources needed for adverse times such as these. And the time of year would be a major factor – winter's long, dark and dreary nights were sure to have a negative impact on people's mental health.

One exception to the lockdown this second time around was that schools were to remain open. The closure of schools in lockdown one meant that I had discontinued the talks I was giving to pupils nation-wide. However, schools were now inviting me again to speak to them. My first Covid-19-era talk was in a school in Dublin at the end of October. I have to admit, it was all a bit strange to begin with – the pupils sat two metres apart, facemasks on, and it was much harder to read the eerily silent room just by the look in pupils' eyes. However, when I opened the floor to some questions, I quickly forget about all of that. I was taken aback and deeply impressed by this young, inquisitive group of teenagers asking me questions on the topic of mental health.

As word spread to other schools that these talks were indeed possi-ble, in the month of November I found myself travelling the length and breadth of the country, spreading my message to more and more bright, inquisitive teenagers. I didn't only talk in schools, but in some businesses too, highlighting the fact that no matter what age you are, your mental health can suffer – I think we have all come to realise that at various stages throughout 2020.

If I were to choose one message to finish with, it would be this: I've seen both sides of the coin – from feeling so low that I thought the only way to stop the pain was to die by suicide, truly believing that the world would be a better place without me; to discovering a path that I hadn't known existed, a path where life is worth living, and worth celebrating. I hope that through my words and actions I can show people that there is a way out of the suffering you may be experiencing. This path, though difficult, is worth travelling.

ACKNOWLEDGEMENTS

Writing this book has been no easy feat, but it has brought me a great sense of pride and achievement. It would not have been possible without my family – my parents Angela and Gerry and my sisters Stephanie, Mairead and Michelle. They were there for me through my bleakest and darkest moments. They were that listening ear, that shoulder to cry on and that guiding hand that led me every step of the way along my path to recovery. Their love and support throughout this entire journey is something I'll be forever grateful for.

Thank you to The O'Brien Press and especially my editor, Eoin O'Brien, who has guided me so brilliantly through this arduous but fulfilling process. They have given me the stage to share my message far and wide, hopefully impacting many along the way.

I want to thank my friends and teammates. Their non-judgmental attitude upon hearing of the inner turmoil I'd been experiencing made my life that bit easier as I began to integrate back into society again. I want to give special mention to my two best friends, Karl and Moe. They stood by my side when I needed them the most, epitomising what best friends are for.

Huge thanks to my mentors and coaches. From everyone at Naomh Mearnóg, who nurtured my raw potential from a very young age and gave me a platform to reach my dreams of playing for Dublin, to everyone associated with Dublin GAA, who made this dream a reality.

To my boss, Philip Duffy, who has been incredibly accommodating, allowing me time off for matches, training sessions, psychologists' appointments, public speaking appearances and writing this book.

To all the staff at St Patrick's mental hospital, and my psychologists Joe Griffin and Dr Francis Valloor. They illuminated a path of hope, a path that I didn't know existed at the beginning of my struggles. They gave me the solid foundation on which I rebuilt my life. They are a major reason why I'm no longer surviving, I'm living.

Also to Dessie Farrell and Mick Galvin, who, with the help of the Gaelic Players Association, made all of this possible.

To all the staff at Dublin City University. A special mention to Michael Kennedy, Enda Fitzpatrick and Niall Moyna, who made my transition into third level seamless, going above and beyond the call of duty, making my life a lot easier when it came to academics, sport and general college life.

And to many others who have had a profound impact on where I am today. Thanks to you all, I have learned to love life again.

Other Books from The O'Brien Press

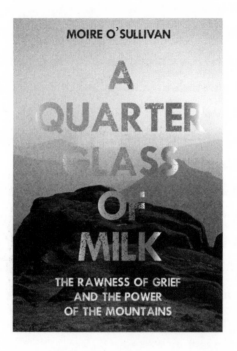

When Moire O'Sullivan's husband, Pete, took his own life, she was left with a stark choice: to weep forever over the glass of milk that had just spilt or get on with the quarter that was still remaining.

As Moire charts the first harrowing year after Pete's death – the shock, the loneliness and the difficulties of single parenting two young children – she also experiences glimpses of hope and acceptance as she trains to become a mountain leader.

A raw and insightful story of grief and renewal.